Do YOU want to live to be 100?

AN EVIDENCE BASED APPROACH TO MAXIMIZING THE LENGTH AND QUALITY OF YOUR LIFE.

(The sooner you start the better!)

DR STEPHEN K FAIRLEY

ISBN: 1470023407

ISBN 13: 9781470023409

Dedication

This book aims to give you the best chance to live a long and healthy life, to make the most of all life offers you. There are no guarantees in the real world however.

I dedicate this book to my very dear friend, Joy, who did everything right. She was never overweight; she exercised, adhered to a healthy diet, loved everyone, and loved life itself. She took on the challenges in life most would run from, such as dealing with other people's difficult children and teenagers as a teacher and psychologist, and setting them on the right track. She did this with one simple tool, love—perhaps the only thing that works. She always gave 110 percent of herself to others in this, and in other tasks, achieved great results. Everyone who met her adored her.

Despite this, cancer struck her down while in her prime. If she had a message for all of you, it would be to treasure life itself, do not take things or other people for granted. Live your life to the fullest.

There are no guarantees.

To JD, first editor of this book and an inspiration in my life.

About the Author

Stephen Fairley is a Medical Specialist in Gastroenterology and Liver disease with a particular interest in fatty liver disease and the metabolic syndrome. He works part time in public practice at the Townsville Hospital and part time in private practice. He is a Clinical Senior Lecturer in the Department of Medicine, James Cook University, Townsville Australia, and has more than twenty years of experience in specialist practice and teaching in Townsville, where he lives with his wife, Carol, and their four children.

Contents

INTRODUCTION

WHEN YOU WERE born life dealt you a hand of cards. Some of these you have no control over and they include things such as your genes, which code for the color of your skin, the color of your eyes, or your potentially achievable height. Genes also code for your genetically predetermined likelihood of developing some diseases including obesity, diabetes, high blood pressure, and a host of other medical conditions. You cannot change the color of your eyes or your skin, but you *can* change the likelihood of developing many diseases. Life is not fair; you may be more likely to get certain diseases than someone else may, but this does not paralyze you, you just have to work harder at it than they do to reverse this outcome and stay well.

You have been born into a time of ever-reducing need for exercise in routine daily activities and perhaps ever-reducing time for exercise in a busy lifestyle. You have been born into a time of increasing availability of high-calorie, nutrient-poor food where food retailers even include toys with unhealthy food to encourage you to buy it for yourself or your children.

"A burger with sugar sweetened bun, potato fries, soft drink *and* a model air plane"," or "carrot sticks and a glass of milk?" Which would you choose as a five-year-old? Which would you choose as a fifty-year-old? You are being swept along in a strong current, and you have the choice of sitting back and saying, "none of this is my fault", "I didn't ask to be born at this time," and "I didn't ask for these genes." You thus go along with societies' norms, as would a pack of sheep, swept by the current and take what comes. Very few people do escape the current—look around you.

The position you currently find yourself in is arguably not your fault. You change nothing, however, by dwelling on this, making excuses, or deciding who or what is to blame for your current medical state. You cannot change the past. You *can* change the future. It is what you make it, and *you* are ultimately responsible for where you end up.

You *do* have the option to fight back. You do not need to accept the sheep mentality. "This is wrong, I can change my life, and I can choose to live a longer healthier life". "I can do this!" Do not let the current of societies' norms sweep you along. Change course and swim out of the current. Be different. It is your choice. Did you ever stop to think that the current you are in might be heading toward a waterfall?

You are likely to find parts of this book and the arguments given in it blunt, rude, and offensive. If they make you angry and emotional, that is good. If so, they are much more likely to make you think critically about your behavior and result in change. Stop and think why they make you angry. The weakest and easiest thing to do is to stop reading.

As a busy practicing medical practitioner, I see patients on a daily basis who want help with their medical conditions. As doctors, we do our best to help patients; however, it is very frustrating that in most cases the people who are most able to help the patients are the patients themselves! Getting this message across is very difficult in our society of "easy fixes," which require minimal input by patients. They have a lot of difficulty accepting any responsibility for their current state and are far from wanting to engage in significant effort to correct it.

The fact is, most western diseases such as obesity, high blood pressure, heart disease, diabetes, and high cholesterol, do not require lifelong medication in most cases. They can be controlled or prevented with lifestyle changes. Likewise, you can prevent many cancers, such as breast, bowel, and pancreas. The sooner these changes are undertaken the better. This book provides you with evidence-based strategies to achieve these goals including options to achieve long-term sustainable weight loss without surgery or fad diets. It may also stop you from ending up on numerous tablets and being dependent on doctors for the rest of your prematurely shortened life. It is direct, honest, and to the point, and I state again, I make no apology if you find some of it offensive or confronting. Do you think this may be because you refuse to take responsibility for your own health issues?

A fifty-five-year-old friend of mine, George, is a great guy, full of life and concerned about the welfare of others. When it comes to his health, he doesn't have a clue. He is what I would describe as lacking insight, happy to leave his head stuck in the sand.

He leaves it all to his doctor. He drifts along with the current, oblivious to what lies ahead.

He plays golf several times per week and walks for exercise when the weather is not too cold. He is happy doing everything he thinks he needs to remain fit and healthy. When we went on a ski holiday recently our Condo was about 120 meters (350 feet) from the lifts, which were up a very slight hill. It took about three to four minutes to walk to the lifts each the morning. Not for George mind you. He was very happy to wait twenty minutes for the bus. "I'll tell you, there is no way I'm going to walk when a perfectly good bus drives right past our front door!" he would say.

He has high cholesterol, borderline diabetes, and borderline high blood pressure. His abdomen is about what a woman could expect at four to five months into a pregnancy

"It is all OK," he assures us. "My doctor says I am not overweight on the basis of my BMI, and I ticked all the right boxes on my last physical." BMI stands for body mass index, which I will define later in the book. He is quite sure he does not have a problem.

Well, wake up George! Your doctor is not being fully truthful. He has told you only what you wanted to hear. He is either a gutless wonder, or he is not really interested in your long-term health prospects; he just wanted you to get out the door so he could move on to the next patient.

Like many primary care givers, he is burned out from trying thousands of times to make people change their ways; almost always, he and his colleagues know they may as well be talking to a brick wall. I can tell you, it is often emotionally exhausting, usually resulting in a pointless emotionally charged, long consultation, with no positive outcome. On top of this is concern for the doctors that they may chase away patients on whom they de-pend for their livelihood. So why should they bother? They tell you what you want to hear so you will come back and see them again. They tell themselves, "Perhaps I will try to address this important issue next time," but they never do. They never have the time; they never have the required energy.

I don't just tell people what they want to hear. I try to put things in clear unambiguous terms. As a result, I have earned the unfortunate nickname "the flying mallet" from some of my colleagues. I'm sure George would agree with them. I find if you shock and offend patients, rather than passively agreeing with them, you are much more likely to get a result. Sure, you may offend many people. I have been called many things, including "Arse hole" for daring to suggest—very politely, I thought—to a particular woman that she should take some responsibility for her current health issues.

If 10 percent of people doctors see as patients take notice of the advice, it is better than 2 percent, and I think 2 percent is being generous for the passive, pleasant approach of George's local doctor. It is easy to see why George's local doctor and almost all his colleagues in this situation behave the way they do. The issue is just too hard to confront. The truth hurts too much, and doctors are sick of being slapped in the face for daring to suggest the truth to their patients. Lucky for you, my face is made of cast iron not soft butter. I'll tell you the truth whether you like it or not.

It will only be a matter of time before George—if he continues on his current path—develops full-blown diabetes and high blood pressure and then needs his chest split open for his coronary artery bypass surgery. Alternatively, he may simply drop dead from his first heart attack or develop a cancer. I would not give him more than five years before one of these events occur.

Do you know someone like George? Does this description fit you?

Just because this is what all your mates do at this age does not mean it is normal. It is a lifestyle choice. At the risk of repeating myself, you do not have to conform to the norms of western society in the twenty-first century and collect all the applicable diseases on the journey. You can avoid most of these conditions. It is up to you. If you want your doctor or someone else to do it all for you; if you don't think you can make an effort yourself; don't bother to read any further—you are wasting your time.

The length of your life is not predetermined at your birth. It is clear that genetic influences are important, but the environment you live in is arguably more so. As discussed, there is also very little you can do about your genes at present (this may change in the future), but you do have control over many other factors. The things you eat, drink, breathe, and take as tablets or supplements; how much exercise you do; your emotional wellbeing; how much sleep you get; and other factors may have a major impact on the length and quality of your life.

There is no such thing as dying from "natural causes." We all die from something and you can avoid or significantly delay many of these things.

In a western society, the commonest causes of death are vascular disease (blood vessels and heart) and cancer. Cancer is not something we invented in the last few hundred years as a consequence of "modern living." It has been around since the dawn of life and in some ways is a consequence of life, with errors in cell division as life regenerates. It matters not if you are a person, a rabbit, a bird, or a dog, about one-third of us will die of cancer of some form. It matters not whether you were born in 2000 BC or AD 2000, you are still at risk.

That is not to imply you do not have a say!

It is up to you to decide if you want to delay or prevent both cancer and heart disease.

There are multiple, evidence-based strategies you can use to alter your own mortality and morbidity. Morbidity refers to diseases altering the quality of your life without killing you (immediately), such as diabetes, obesity, high blood pressure, arthritis, heart attacks, strokes, and dementia.

I base this book on evidence I took from high-quality studies in medical and scientific literature. I am not a believer in magical hocus pocus, such as iridology (reading the iris of your eye) or astrology (studying the stars). Remember just because something is natural does not mean it is good for you. I do not usually prescribe arsenic or cyanide for my patients; however, these substances abound in nature.

As a gastroenterologist, I have seen a number of people die or need liver transplantation after taking "natural" Chinese herbal remedies and tonics, which patients perceive as safe. Just because someone tells you it is natural doesn't mean it cannot kill you, and it certainly doesn't mean it will necessarily do you any good. It is likely to cost you a lot of money, however.

Our quest for evidence-based answers is something constantly evolving. We don't have all the answers yet. We are finding new information and "truths" all the time, sometimes reversing previous beliefs or "truths." The scientific community has in the past taken as fact that the world is flat or that flight is impossible, and clearly, these views are not correct. The broader scientific community has become much more careful about what they consider evidence; however, we still get it wrong from time to time. The evidence quoted in this book is as up to date as possible at the time of the books' publication.

We'll review many factors including lifestyle, diet, supplements, and medication. I will clarify these issues based on the evidence available.

- Will they do you any good?

- Will they do you any harm?

- How much is too much?

- Should you be taking this? Why? What is the evidence?

References will allow those of you who want to check the scientific publications to do so yourselves.

GRADING OF EVIDENCE:

There are numerous ways of critically assessing the level of evidence for a recommendation or finding in the scientific literature, and I will touch on this topic from time to time in discussion to reinforce it. At the risk of boring the readers, you do need to be critical of what you read and what others tell you, and I will use four levels of evidence as a rough guide. These run from worst to best:

LEVEL FOUR

'Expert' opinion:

"Echinacea cures the common cold"

Heard this before?

This is the lowest level of evidence and frequently wrong so be careful what people (including your doctor) suggest unless backed up by other evidence.

LEVEL THREE

Case reports:

For example, "I treated three people with Echinacea for the common cold, and they all got better!"

"Wow! It must be wonderful stuff. Where can I get some?"

Therefore, should all people take it whenever they get a cold? Would the opinion of the person trying to sell it to you be influenced by the fact they would make personal profit from the sale? Has your pharmacist or naturopath recommended this to you recently?

Could it be they were all going to get better anyway? All you can really conclude here is "at least the Echinacea didn't kill me."

LEVEL TWO:

Comparison studies:

Level two evidence attempts to compare two groups together: those who take Echinacea, for example, with those who do not. This type of study is a case-control, cohort, or observational study where one group has a factor such as exercise, or Echinacea, and another group does not. The problem is there are many other factors not taken into account that cannot be effectively "controlled for." If you compare a group taking Echinacea with a group not taking this for the common cold, there may be many reasons for an apparent difference in the outcome. Those taking the Echinacea may be a very different group who are younger, health conscious, have a healthy diet, exercise regularly, and take other medications compared with overweight "couch potatoes" who are at higher risk of chest infection and make no effort with respect to their health.

There is also an effect called the placebo effect. This is very real, very potent, and very much under-utilized by conventional medical or health practitioners. Non-conventional health practitioners probably overuse this; however, I do not have a problem with this as long as it does the patient good. The placebo effect says essentially that if you believe in the person telling you something and you believe what you are given is going to do you good, it will. This is the power of the mind making you better, and I state again it is very real and can be very powerful—it is not "all in your head." This effect is best seen in conditions such as irritable bowel syndrome (IBS) where patients complain of abdominal pain, bloating, and variable bowel habit. If given a placebo sugar tablet—which patients are told will help them—and they believe in their treating physicians, it will help with up to 70 percent of patients with irritable bowel syndrome reporting they get a benefit from the medication. Perhaps as much as 20 percent of the population has mild symptoms of IBS.

No, it doesn't mean the patients are mad; they are normal human beings like you and me. It simply means positive thought is a powerful healer.

LEVEL ONE:

This is the best you can get.

It makes an attempt to *randomize* the two groups without any bias about who is treated and who is not.

It attempts to *control* for variables between the two groups so they are both the same age, sex, and weight and have the same other habits, such as drinking or smoking that may affect the outcome.

It attempts to be *double-blind,* meaning that neither the patient nor the investigator running the study know who is getting the active treatment and who is getting the "sugar pill" or *placebo*—hopefully avoiding the placebo effect on the patient and bias of interpretation of results by the investigator.

It moves forward in time or is *prospective,* allowing the investigator to watch for other factors that may upset the results as opposed to guessing what may have happened in the past in a retrospective study—looking back in time such as an observational study.

Hence the term *"prospective, randomized, double-blind placebo-controlled study."*

You can go one better than this with a *meta-analysis,* where numerous similar studies are combined and looked at together. This makes the study more powerful statistically.

I use the term "attempts" in describing the above study type, as nothing is perfect and studies do not always go as planned. Some studies are much better done and designed than others.

If you are interested, the most recent prospective, randomized, double-blind, placebo-controlled study found that Echinacea is not of any use for the common cold, despite earlier lower-quality evidence suggesting it was effective. Read it yourself; don't waste your money.

Bruce Barrett et al. Echinacea for Treating the Common Cold. Annals of Internal Medicine, December 20, 2010 vol. 153 no. 12 769-777

So does this all really matter?

Well yes it does. Let me give you a real life example of "expert opinion."

Before I do so, however, let me make the point for those of you who already feel I dislike non-western or natural forms of healing or medicine. This is not the case, I am very much in favor of anything that will do patients good, and I and many of my colleagues in the western and natural medicine areas have been striving for this for years. I will give examples of many natural therapies that are effective in the text to follow.

What I have a problem with is natural or other practitioners harming patients or tricking them into handing over large quantities of money for effectively nothing or for the privilege of experiencing harm by their treatment. Hopefully this type of behavior applies to the minority of the natural or western medical practitioners out there offering their services to you.

Several years ago, I began seeing multiple patients for colonoscopy (to examine their large bowel) because a local naturopath iridologist was looking at the iris of the eye (colored part) for a general checkup and proclaiming, "Goodness me! You have a bowel cancer! It is all right, however, because it looks to be in the early stages, and if you take this medicine, hopefully, we can cure the cancer. Thank goodness you came to be examined today!"

The naturopath gave the patients a small bottle of liquid and a dropper and told to take three drops four times a day for the next six weeks. The special medication was very expensive at $650;

however, they were told, "This is really very cheap considering it will save your life!"

The naturopath then got the patients back and re-examined their eyes in six weeks and proclaimed, "It is OK we got it in time, you are cured!"

As you can imagine, some of the patients were skeptical and came to me to have their bowel examined. I might add that the six patients I saw—all with the same story—had all bought the liquid and were taking it. The naturopath was a good salesperson. With such a serious potential problem, the patients obviously thought they should have a bet each way!

One of the patients let me have the fluid analyzed, and it was just salt water or sodium chloride. Not one of the six patients examined had even a tiny polyp (very early change, which could become a cancer), the colonoscopies were all entirely normal. They had only just begun their "therapy." How many of these patients did not come to see me? I was probably only aware of the tip of the iceberg here.

Worse still, working in my field where cancer is common, I frequently see patients talked out of conventional, potentially curative treatment by their naturopath or family members. They are told to try brand new natural or alternative therapies that the naturopathic and nutritional communities tout as 100 percent effective with no harmful side effects.

As far as I am aware, all these patients (I have lost count of how many) have died, and I am still waiting to see one survive, but I am not holding my breath. This does not apply to those lacking in education or intelligence who you may feel can easily have the wool pulled over their eyes by a good sales pitch. The brightest and most creative in our society are also at risk. Have you read about how one of the founders of Apple computers managed his pancreatic cancer?

This is why an evidence-based approach is so important.

This is why some doctors feel so strongly about these issues.

Be careful of "expert opinion" with nothing but hot air to back it up. The "expert" would probably make a good used-car salesperson too.

CHAPTER 1

Preventable Disease in Western Society: An Overview of Why Most of Us Will Die Younger than We Need To.

The Metabolic Syndrome

THE METABOLIC SYNDROME is the reason we are likely to be the first generation in several hundred years to die younger than our parents did. This syndrome is strongly linked to obesity and is rapidly becoming a global health issue as obesity becomes more and more common. As of 2008, in the USA 68 percent of men and 72 percent of women are either overweight or obese.

The metabolic syndrome is a relatively recent term, which I describe as an exercise-deficiency state. A medical perspective defines it as the combination of obesity around the trunk with high blood pressure, raised bad fats and cholesterol in the bloodstream, and the key ingredient and initial problem of insulin resistance. Insulin resistance is a term used to describe the body becoming less sensitive to insulin, with rising insulin levels necessary to keep the blood sugar in the normal range. You could consider this the result of it all being soaked up by the excessive fat in the body, as body fat consumes a large amount of insulin and a person reaches the point where there is simply not enough to go around. The fat also produces substances that interfere with the action of insulin—so called "insulin antagonists."

FATTY LIVER DISEASE

The liver is one of the first organs affected in this process, which involves the entire body. One of insulin's strongest actions is to push blood sugar or glucose into cells, and the liver cells take far more than most. This causes fatty liver disease because the sugar turns into fat, causing the liver cells to fill with fat or cause "fatty liver." I stress this is *not*, as some authors would have you believe, a disease primarily of the liver. Your liver does *not* need to be "cleansed" with expensive dietary supplements or special diets, so please do not waste your time and money. It is simply a consequence of running out of space to store nutrients, in this case sugar, which is stored as fat. Energy can be more efficiently stored as fat than sugar, so the liver converts the sugar to fat for this reason. Fatty liver disease is primarily a result of excess carbohydrate (sugar) intake and not of fat intake, as many believe. It is quite simply a "food overload" situation.

This condition is not just a human disease. Any animal subjected to excessive calorific intake and denied exercise is likely to develop fatty liver. Why do the French put geese in a cage where they cannot exercise and force-feed them with a tube down their throat? Perhaps it has something to do with the fact that a liver filled with fat makes good pate when you mince it up. Perhaps it is just as well you are not a French goose!

Fatty liver disease may also cause liver scarring (cirrhosis) with resultant liver failure and death, or the need for liver transplantation. That's right; you can die from cirrhosis of the liver without a drop of alcohol ever touching your lips. Fatty liver disease is already becoming a very common cause of liver failure. It may be close to overtaking alcohol as the commonest cause in western societies.

Roughly speaking, about half the patients with the serious form of fatty liver disease (nonalcoholic steatohepatitis or NASH) will die from liver failure and the other half from vascular disease or cancer, including liver cancer (hepatoma), which is much more common in the presence of cirrhosis of the liver.

There are two main types of fatty liver disease: That which is associated with inflammation in the liver (NASH) and that without significant inflammation (nonalcoholic fatty liver disease or NAFLD). The significance is if you do not have inflammation, you are less likely to damage your liver over time and less likely to get liver cancer. The remainder of the metabolic syndrome still applies however, lurking in the background, waiting to get you in other ways. The only way to tell the difference for sure is to have your doctor look at some of your liver under the microscope with a liver biopsy. Not something to be undertaken lightly because of potentially life-threatening complications.

How do you move from the early, less serious changes of NAFLD to the later more serious changes of NASH?

That's easy—just increase your weight! It couldn't be simpler.

Step right up! There are many fast food outlets out there ready and waiting to help you achieve this goal. You may even be able to pick up a DVD to watch on the TV while you eat your meal. Now wouldn't that be nice?

So you think I am being a bit harsh, do you? Well, what is your reaction every time you read about some innocent soul killed or maimed in a traffic accident? What would you say if I told you more than a *thousand times* as many ignorant souls die prematurely or are maimed with complications of the metabolic syndrome?

Would your response be, "Could I have another burger, super-sized fries, and a large soft drink to go please?"

Perhaps you should stop reading now.

There is a very strong correlation between the likelihood of having NASH as your underlying type of fatty liver disease and increasing weight.

There do appear to be other factors at play here as well and these include things as diverse as your DNA, the type of bacteria in your colon, if you are a coffee drinker, and so on. Presumably, some bacteria in the colon produce a toxin that causes inflammation in the liver, and some antioxidants such as those in coffee seem to protect your liver. One of the major functions of your liver is to filter out all the bad things or poisons from your gut, a bit like how a charcoal filter on a drinking-water tap filters out chlorine. All the blood coming from the gut (portal system) has to pass through the liver to get to the rest of your body (systemic circulation) and is filtered on the way. This is thought to be one of the reasons you go into a coma (hepatic encephalopathy) in liver failure, as the poisons from your gut get to your brain unfiltered. It may also be the reason some colonic bacteria are more likely to cause liver inflammation than others in the presence of fat in the liver.

DIABETES

There is a limit to how much insulin the pancreas can put out, eventually its blood level will peak, and then the blood sugar starts to rise. At this stage, your doctor tells you, "Congratulations, you have diabetes; you can reduce your estimated life expectancy by about ten years." We term this "type 2" or "maturity onset" diabetes. It is not the same as type 1 diabetes, usually occurring at a much younger age, where the immune system appears to kill off the insulin producing cells in the pancreas causing very low levels of insulin.

You may like to think your newly diagnosed type 2 diabetes is reversible; however, this is usually only the case if you act quickly. Unfortunately, your pancreatic insulin producing cells appear to wear out and die if you keep them running at 150 percent of their capacity to maintain your high insulin levels. After that, you will need to start giving yourself injections of insulin multiple times per day and your diabetes may well be with you for the rest of your prematurely shortened life.

There has never been a time in our history where we have had such an abundance of food and ever-increasing reasons and excuses for doing less exercise. We have existed as a single species for about the last 150,000 years, continuing to develop with evolution where our very existence depended on a considerable amount of physical exertion every day. All of a sudden, particularly in the last fifty to one-hundred years, this need for physical exertion has evaporated for most of us, and multiple new diseases have developed.

As described above, when we are not exercising and have plentiful supplies of food, our bodies store this away for a time when we may not have enough and need to draw on our stores. This is clearly an important survival technique that has developed with evolution; those who could not do this in times of famine died out, as did their genes. Some human races are much better at doing this than others—a point with significant implications for them in terms of developing the metabolic syndrome. They are able to develop the syndrome without being significantly overweight; however, the treatment (exercise) is still the same and is still effective. Sure, there is a genetic component to this disease explaining why some people and some races are more likely to develop it; however, to say "My diabetes is genetic like my father's or mother's, and there is nothing I can do about it" is simply untrue. If you want to live your life making excuses like this to yourself, I would not bother to read any further. There is probably little I can do to help you if you have no interest in helping yourself.

When I discuss obesity in this book, it is the fat on the inside that we term "visceral fat" that matters, not the fat on the outside, which is under the skin or "subcutaneous fat." The visceral fat is in the liver and around the gut, and is the first your body draws on when you begin to lose weight. It is termed very metabolically active. This fat is more quickly laid down by your body and more quickly removed when needed. The fat around your backside and legs, arms, and breasts is not very metabolically active with two consequences. This subcutaneous fat is not as important in the metabolic syndrome and is the last to go with exercise and diet, and as many of you know, it is difficult to remove.

The problem in our society now is that we rarely draw on our energy stores, and our body becomes overloaded with these stores, which alters our metabolic system and our physique, causing a fat abdomen, a liver full of fat, and insulin resistance. Following on from this or at the same time, people usually develop high blood pressure, raised cholesterol, and type 2 diabetes. These then lead to heart disease, strokes, and early cancers to name just a few possibilities. How many tablets does it take to treat all of these conditions? How many are you taking?

Another unfortunate problem associated with the metabolic syndrome is a dramatic increase in some types of cancer in the developed world. The reason for this is not entirely clear, but it may in part relate to something secreted with insulin from the pancreas called "insulin-like growth factor." This is necessary for cell growth but it also promotes the growth of cancer cells. If you double your output of insulin, you will also double your output of insulin-like growth factor and perhaps your risk for developing some cancers.

ARE YOU AT RISK?

Body mass index (BMI) refers to your weight in Kg divided by your height in meters squared. Your height will be on your driver's license. If you were 2 m tall and 100 kg, your BMI would be 25, at the upper limit of normal. Check yours now, is it greater than 25?

18–25 is considered normal

25–30 is considered overweight

>30 is considered obese

An alternative measurement is your waist-hip circumference. Use a tape measure and measure around your mid abdomen at about the level of your umbilicus (belly button) and at the level of your hips, if the first number is greater than the second number, you are at risk. Neither of these are perfect tools; however, they are a useful guide. It is certainly possible to have a normal

BMI and still be overweight for your body type with risk factors for the metabolic syndrome.

VASCULAR DISEASE

Vascular disease refers to disease of the arteries that carry life giving blood and, therefore, oxygen around your body. As you get older, they age along with the rest of you with degenerative changes in the walls of the arteries and the internal lumen clogging up with fat and scar tissue, blocking the flow of blood. This begins as fatty streaks on the inside lining of your arteries in adolescence that become thicker plaques in early adulthood. These then become ulcerated causing blood to clot on their surface blocking the artery in middle-older age. The walls change from being elastic and flexible in young people to inelastic and rigid in older people, with loss of the elastic tissue and deposition of calcium. Eventually with weaker walls or with the internal lumen clogging up, they will break or block up. The consequences depend on where the blood vessels are.

In coronary artery disease, blockage of the arteries in the heart causes heart attacks if it occurs quickly or angina (pain from heart muscle that cannot get enough blood when you exercise), when it occurs slowly. Individuals with the metabolic syndrome are *three times more likely to die from heart disease than healthy counterparts are.*

Arnt Erik Tjonna et al. Aerobic Interval Training Versus continuous Moderate Exercise as a Treatment for the Metabolic Syndrome. Circulation. 2008:118:346-354.

In cerebrovascular disease, disease of the arteries in the brain causes strokes, which can be hemorrhagic if the artery bursts or thrombotic if the artery blocks. The result is much the same and depends on the part of the brain that dies, resulting in, for example, loss of sight, loss of the ability to speak, or loss of muscle function such as moving one side of your body. Individuals with the metabolic syndrome *are one and a half to three times as likely to have a stroke when compared to their healthy counterparts.*

Bernadette Boden-Albala et al. Metabolic Syndrome and Ischemic Stroke Risk. Stroke. 2008;39:30-35

Tatjana Rundek et al. Insulin Resistance and Risk of Ischemic Stroke Among Nondiabetic Individuals From the Northern Manhattan Study. Arch Neurol. 2010 67(10):1195-1200

In peripheral vascular disease, arterial disease occurs in the periphery, such as a leg where an artery may block. If a person does not seek urgent medical intervention, it may cause death of the leg, resulting in the need to amputate the leg to keep the person alive.

The choice you get in all of this is whether you want it to occur sooner, or later. What are the main risk factors for vascular disease that bring it on earlier?

They are high cholesterol, high blood pressure, diabetes, and smoking. Other contributing issues such as being of male sex and of older age you can do little about. The first three factors describe the metabolic syndrome, which I stress yet again is a *lifestyle choice* in the vast majority of cases. Smoking speaks for itself, and if you have a death wish, that is up to you. I would suggest it is likely to be less messy in the long run, to step in front of a train than to smoke yourself to death. I am not thinking only about you but also about the poor souls who are going to have to look after you while you slowly die. How much pain are you prepared to inflict on your family or loved ones? Having offended a number of you, I will say no more about smoking.

The metabolic syndrome markedly accelerates this whole process causing arteries to block much sooner than they otherwise might have done with obvious consequences. Remember there is no such thing as dying of natural causes. We all die of something, you just get a say as to whether you would like this to occur sooner, or later.

CANCER

This is often an unfortunate consequence of the metabolic syndrome.

As I have previously mentioned, cancer is part of life; it is not something new we invented in the last century, as many seem to believe. Even discussing it makes people anxious because of the perception we can do very little about it, and it is likely to be a death sentence—perhaps a slow and painful one.

Fortunately, it is unlikely this is going to be the case forever, and we are getting better and better at understanding how reproduction at a cellular level works and what controls it. Hopefully this means we will soon be able to intervene effectively.

It is the loss of these controls of cellular division that cause uncontrolled cellular division, which we term cancer. The same thing can happen when cells fail to die when they have done their job, and consequently the body eventually fills up with them, blocking normal body functions. For example, with some blood cell cancers where cells fail to die off when they have done their job, the excess cells clog up the bone marrow so you cannot make blood anymore. These cells do not necessarily divide in a rapid uncontrolled fashion, they have just lost the ability to die off after use, and you eventually run out of places to store them. Most cancers are a combination of these two processes. The cells in your body either, fail to die off, or they undergo uncontrolled division.

The thing that controls this cellular division and cellular death (which we term apoptosis) is the DNA (deoxyribonucleic acid) in the cellular nucleus. The DNA is the code from which you are assembled—the plans from which you were built—and is unique, perhaps excepting identical twins. The DNA has numerous functions controlling cellular division and in repairing errors, which may occur with the division. Damage to DNA that controls cell division may then result in loss of this control and subsequent cancer. This may occur by chance with a cell that is dividing making an error or because of external things that damage DNA. The things that may damage DNA include some chemical substances or radiation, both of which we are exposed to every day no matter where we live. High doses of DNA dam-aging chemicals or radiation, however, make cancer much more likely to occur.

What else contributes to your risk of dying from cancer? Could it be something over which you have control? You guessed it— the metabolic syndrome is a big player in the incidence of many western cancers. Some studies show bowel cancer, for example, has increased by up to 3.4 times.

Edward Giovannucci et al. Physical Activity, Obesity, and Risk for Colon Cancer and Adenoma in Men. March 1, 1995 vol. 122 no. 5 327-334 Annals of internal medicine)

The risk of breast cancer also increased, especially in postmeno-pausal women.

B.A.Stoll. Breast cancer: the obesity connection. Br J Cancer. 1994 May; 69(5): 799–801

Other sites of cancer associated with increased risk in the meta-bolic syndrome include the cervix, uterus, prostate, pancreas, liver, kidney, and oesophagus.

Stephanie Cowey and Robert Hardy. The Metabolic Syndrome. A High-Risk state for Cancer? Am J Pathol. 2006, Nov;169(5):1505-1522.

OTHER CONDITIONS ASSOCIATED WITH THE METABOLIC SYNDROME

Polycystic ovarian syndrome (PCOS) is where women may develop male features with their obesity, such as markedly increased body hair, acne, and a deeper voice, as well as irregular periods and infertility.

These women have increased levels of male hormones and multiple cysts in the ovaries as the name suggests. The cause of PCOS is not fully understood and there are clearly genetic influences as in the metabolic syndrome. Some of the increased male hormones may be made in the periphery in fat, converting female like hormones to male hormones. One thing is certain however, as weight increases, the risk for developing PCOS increases, and the disease is strongly associated with the metabolic syndrome.

Kidney failure is an important complication of the metabolic syndrome both to the individual and to the costs imposed on society as a whole.

The small filters in the kidney (glomeruli) get damaged, with one of the earliest findings being leakage of protein in the urine. They may eventually fill up and block with this protein-type material, at which time your kidneys fail. The result is death from kidney failure or alternatively you can go on a dialysis machine to filter your blood every three days. If you are lucky, you may be able to get hold of someone else's kidney (that they have not destroyed by their lifestyle) for kidney transplantation, but life will never again be the same. To stop your body rejecting the new kidney you will need many drugs with many side effects including a higher risk of developing some cancers,, such as skin cancer and lymphoma.

Perhaps you should get your doctor to check your urine with a simple dipstick to see if you have protein in it as several drugs do slow the loss of kidney function if begun early and delay the need for dialysis. Better still, perhaps you should start exercising now and prevent the syndrome in the first place?

Obstructive sleep apnea (OSA) is when every time you try to sleep you obstruct your upper airway and partially wake up, never getting a restful or effective night's sleep. You do not fully recover consciousness and may have no idea that you are getting a poor night's sleep. Your partner may complain you snore a lot or even witness numerous episodes of you stopping breathing (apnea) during the night. The result is marked daytime tiredness, lethargy, and other medical problems, such as high blood pressure. These problems cease by correcting the sleep apnea, and typically, those with sleep apnea say they have not felt so well in years after effective treatment. This usually involves wearing a tight mask over the face at night and some people cannot tolerate this. Many factors may contribute to OSA, but obesity is by far the best documented. As you increase your BMI or your waist hip circumference, your likelihood for having sleep apnea progressively increases with other potentially serious health issues, including the chance of dying or killing someone else in a motor vehicle accident should you fall asleep at the wheel.

The nonmedical cost to the community from factors such as road traffic accidents or poor performance at work are huge and difficult to calculate.

Have you been feeling tired lately?

Raised uric acid levels in the blood may cause gout (painful arthritis) and kidney stones.

CHAPTER 2

What You Can Do To Avoid Dying Prematurely; the Factors Affecting the Length and Quality of Your Life.

The metabolic syndrome may be very much more common now than it was in the past but was recognized by physicians even before the birth of Christ.

"If we could give every individual the right amount of nourishment and exercise, not too little and not too much, we would have found the safest way to health." Hippocrates, 460-377 BC

Exercise

"But doctor, I exercise almost every day! I almost exercised on Monday, I almost exercised on Tuesday, I almost exercised on Wednesday…"

Sound familiar?

If you want to fix a problem most effectively, you start at the beginning before it even occurs and prevent it happening.

This should be our aim as a society and where we direct our resources. The sad situation, however, is that this disease, the metabolic syndrome, has already taken hold of a large number of people in the developed world and is slowly killing them. Our governments direct many billions of health care dollars at the end result, with relatively ineffective "band aids," such as blood pressure tablets, rather than directing them at *primary prevention,* thus preventing the associated diseases such as high blood pressure from occurring in the first place.

There are many hundreds of articles in the medical literature showing that exercise largely prevents or cures the metabolic syndrome or its components.

It has been shown in Animal models and in Human studies that exercise reverses the primary problem of insulin resistance with normalization of blood sugar and insulin levels, curing diabetes if begun early.

Exercise has also been shown to reduce blood pressure, to reduce the bad fats (triglycerides) and the bad cholesterol levels (low-density lipoprotein or LDL), to increase the good or protective cholesterol (high-density lipoprotein or HDL), and to remove all fat from the liver. As a consequence of this, your risk of dying from a heart attack is more than halved by regular moderate exercise.

Rozenn N. Lemaitre. Lesure-Time physical Activity and the Risk of Primary Cardiac Arrest. Arch Intern Med. 1999;159(7):686

This effect in reduction of cardiovascular disease is not related to your age, your sex, or your ethnic background, so stop looking for excuses!

Marie Cooney et al.Risk Prediction in cardiovascular Medicine Circulation. 2010;122(7):743

You do not have to be thin to get this effect. If you look at sumo wrestlers in Japan, when they are training, they have no fat in the liver and no insulin resistance despite the fact we would term them obese. As soon as they stop training, their livers fill with fat and their insulin levels rise, and this occurs within days to weeks.

WHAT TYPE OF EXERCISE?

We do not yet have all the answers here; however, *any* exercise is good with respect to the metabolic syndrome and, within reason, the more the better. If you already exercise then you are deserving of a round of applause.

There are many different ways of exercising. A few of these they include:

Moderate continuous exercise where you aim to get your heart rate to 70 percent of the predicted safe maximum for your age. This safe maximum roughly calculates as 220 minus your age.

Aerobic interval training where you train in short bursts getting your heart rate to 90 percent of your predicted safe maximum.

Physical strength training where the primary aim is strengthening muscles as opposed to cardiac and respiratory fitness.

There does appear to be some evidence that exercising harder, as in the aerobic interval training, is associated with more improvement in features of the metabolic syndrome, such as insulin resistance, than the other two options listed. In these comparison studies, the time spent exercising was the same in each.

You may be interested to know that studies have shown this to be the case with rats and humans who have the metabolic syndrome.

Have you been craving cheese lately?

Per Magnus Haram. Aerobic Interval training vs. continuous moderate exercise in the metabolic syndrome of rats artificially selected for low aerobic capacity. Cardiovascular Research (81)4 723-732

Arnt Erik Tjonna et al. Aerobic Interval Training Versus Continuous Moderate Exercise as a Treatment for the Metabolic Syndrome. Circulation. 2008 118:346-354.

HOW MUCH EXERCISE DO I HAVE TO DO?

Well, ideally enough to correct the metabolic syndrome, which in my experience is generally a lot more than most patients think. As a general guide, however, thirty minutes of brisk walking daily is what is recommended; however, as mentioned above this may not be the ideal form of exercise to tackle the metabolic syndrome; more intense and longer exercise periods may be more beneficial.

You should check with your doctor however, especially if you have features of the metabolic syndrome to ensure what you are planning to do is safe. Start gradually, not running a 42 km marathon on your first day of the new exercise program. If you do have underlying heart disease, which you may have no idea about, it is even more important for you to start exercising but preferably not by dropping dead from a heart attack on day one.

I DO NOT HAVE TIME TO EXERCISE!

Don't bother telling me this, I have heard it all before—thousands of times while trying to educate patients about these issues. You are wasting your breath and my time. I like to practice what I preach. I work in a relatively small community for a medical specialist, with about 200,000 people. We are under-resourced in terms of gastroenterologists (my specialty). As a result, my usual day is ten to fourteen hours long away from home and includes several hours at home doing paperwork each night. I have to get up at five o'clock to get in an hour's aerobic exercise before going to work and have been doing so for the last fifteen years. I am not trying to boast, just make a point. I am nothing special, (just ask my wife!); if I can do this so can you. Hopefully you will have more sense than to work the hours I do and *do* have time to exercise, so cut out the crap, and get on with it!

Do you watch the day's news on TV at night? Do you sit on the couch to do this? Well get rid of the couch and put your exercise bike in front the TV. When you finish the news, you should need to take a shower and change your sweaty clothes. Remember your heart rate has to be at least 70 percent of your predicted maximum, so get yourself a heart monitor as well. All sport stores have them. You are not on the bike for a pleasant chat with your partner; you can do that with your evening meal.

Do you have trouble sleeping at night and consequently feel you couldn't possibly survive with any less sleep? You might be surprised the quality of your sleep is, within reason, more important than the quantity. How could you improve the quality of your sleep? Could it be by exercising in the evening?

Am I a bit tough in my approach?

Well I can tell you after nearly thirty years of practicing medicine I know that pussyfooting around and pandering to your excuses (most of which I am sorry to say I would class as pathetic) does *not* achieve results. The cold, hard truth often does. Most patients do actually want the truth even if it makes them grimace.

Don't bother making the excuses, your time would be better spent planning to be one of the youngest or largest residents in the local cemetery. And while you are at it, get them to put "this person didn't have time to exercise" on your gravestone as a sobering message to others.

This is not to say that weight loss is not important, and this or exercise (preferably both) will cure the metabolic syndrome in the vast majority of cases.

Weight loss / diet

The best evidence for curing the syndrome by weight loss alone comes from many studies of patients after bariatric (weight loss) surgery, where the stomach may be bypassed or reduced in size surgically. The results of these studies have shown repeatedly that weight loss can cure all the features of the metabolic syndrome. As discussed already the sooner you intervene the better, and the more effective the surgery the more likely you are to experience a cure.
Obesity is a large risk factor for the metabolic syndrome as is well documented in mountains of medical literature.

In the Framingham heart study the incidence of the metabolic syndrome was:

Five percent in participants with a normal weight
Twenty-two percent if overweight (BMI of 25–30)
Sixty percent if obese (BMI of >30)
What was your BMI?

The Framingham heart study, initially from Framingham Massachusetts, refers to following large groups of normal, well people over time to see who gets heart or other diseases and then calculating risk factors for these diseases. It has been going since 1948 and has contributed a lot to our understanding of the risk factors for heart and vascular disease, and involves tens of thousands of volunteers.

In a study of laparoscopic gastric bypass surgery involving fifty-three patients, thirty-two of the patients (60 percent) had the metabolic syndrome before surgery. Twelve months after surgery only one patient (2 percent) still had the syndrome. On average, they had lost 78 percent of their excess body fat. There is no question that surgery works; however, it is expensive, can be dangerous, and is not without side effects. You are likely to live longer, however, with surgery than without if you cannot lose weight by other means.

Atul Madan et al. Metabolic syndrome: yet another co-morbidity gastric bypass helps cure. Surgery for Obesity, Volume 2, Issue 1, pages 48-51, January 2006

There is nothing magical about weight loss; however, it is very difficult for most people, and there are other factors at play here you may not have heard about. Put simply, it is a case of more fuel/food put in to your body than you are able to burn or take out. Your solution is either to put less in (diet) or take more out (exercise).

If you achieve this, you will lose weight. If you feel you are already dieting and nothing is happening, you are still eating more than your body needs, whatever your dietician or your defense mechanisms may tell you. I have lost count of how many obese patients have told me, "I eat nothing doctor, and I cannot lose any weight!" They have my sympathy, as I know the task is very difficult; however, my usual response is to ask how many obese prisoners of war they saw in the horrific pictures of the POWs coming out of Japanese concentration camps after WWII. Sometimes, unfortunately, confronting patients with the unsavory and shocking truth is the only way to get a point across effectively, especially if trying to change their behavior. It is exceedingly unlikely you have a "disease" that makes weight loss more difficult for you than other people.

The difficulty in weight loss comes with the body's own control mechanisms. If you try to lose weight by eating less your brain's inbuilt protective mechanisms increase your appetite and reduce your metabolic rate to make it much harder for you. Your brain has set your body's ideal weight too high, and it is going to fight you all the way, by stimulating your appetite. Your body's idea of your ideal weight may once have been ideal; however, over the years of not enough exercise and too many calories it has gradually pushed up and up, probably by only a few kilograms or pounds per year. Then when you decide to go on a diet, your body's protective mechanisms step into play and increase your appetite. You may be surprised to know your body will also resist attempts to increase your weight by turning off your appetite and burning off extra calories; however, we often defeat this mechanism by shear persistence with a very high calorie intake and time, gradually pushing up your body's settings for your ideal weight. It would be easy if we knew how to control this inbuilt mechanism, and I am sure an effective safe pill will come one day, but it is not here yet. It may come too late for you, so *stop* waiting for it.

There are some very important principles here to avoid the increased appetite that is causing you to fail. One of the most important is to recognize what it is in food that switches off your appetite. Of the three main classes of food (protein, carbohydrate, and fat), it is the protein that is most effective at making you feel full. If you eat a large serving of meat or fish, which are largely protein, you are likely to feel full and be able to stop. If you eat a large serving of fried potato chips, which are fat and carbohydrate, you will simply keep eating until you cannot physically fit any more in your stomach and, as a result, get twice as many calories. I know I find it hard to stop eating potato fries. No stop signal comes through from the brain with carbohydrate and only a small signal with fat. If you take a high protein drink—for example, whey protein readily available from the chemist or gym—fifteen to thirty minutes before your meal, you will feel full and find it easier to have a smaller meal. Try it.

Using smaller plates has also helped aid in weight loss, and I would suggest you seriously consider changing your crockery if you are serious about weight loss. This will limit your serving size, but you will have to limit the number of servings you take.

For decades, experts told us the bad foods were high cholesterol and high animal fat foods, such as eggs and red meat, and we should avoid them because they cause heart disease. Well there may be a small amount of truth to this; however, the real enemy of weight loss in modern society is carbohydrate and not fat. Some fats, such as fish oil, are very protective for heart disease. They are also more effective at turning off your appetite than carbohydrates are, but do contain more calories per gram (nine calories per gram for fat and four calories per gram for carbohydrate).

Carbohydrate refers to simple sugars such as sucrose (cane sugar) or fructose (fruit sugar) and to long chains of sugars joined together, which are called complex carbohydrates. Examples of these include grains such as wheat or rice and vegetables such as potatoes or pumpkin. Another form of carbohydrate you are all familiar with is fiber, which by definition we cannot digest ourselves; however, the bacteria in our bowel often can, and they may provide a small source of calories. Carbohydrate is the main fuel for our bodies. Many processed foods contain it in huge amounts. Do you know how many teaspoons of sugar there are in a 750 ml bottle of soft drink? It is about twenty-six. Have you ever tried to eat twenty-six teaspoons of sugar? I doubt many of us would be able to. It is easy to drink a bottle of coke when you are thirsty, however.

An imbalance between energy input and lack of exercise or energy output causes, at least in large part, the metabolic syndrome. As mentioned earlier, the cure is to tackle either end of this equation. Your choice—either take less in or put more out.

Now if you think exercising is an easy way to lose weight you are seriously mistaken. It is likely to increase your appetite, and on its own is likely to disappoint you. You can do a large amount of exercise on very few calories. Two slices of bread, for example, give you approximately enough energy/calories to walk up fifty stories of a skyscraper. The implications are you need to do this much exercise to get back to where you started before eating the bread, without losing any weight at all. It is much easier on you, and your knees, to not eat it in the first place.

Generally speaking, you burn more calories when you are sleeping in bed than doing your daily exercise program. This is not to put you off exercise, just to keep things in context: the way to lose weight effectively is to eat less, not to exercise madly and disregard your food intake. I cannot stress enough how important it is you understand this concept if you wish to be successful.

I don't mean to imply that exercise is not potentially helpful with weight loss; however, the primary mechanism here is probably increased muscle bulk, not burning calories when you exercise. Muscle is much more expensive in terms of calories to run and keep alive than fat. Fat literally just sits there and needs very little care. Muscle, however, is constantly burning calories and takes glucose and fatty acids (calories) from the blood stream just to keep itself alive. The obvious implication is that if you exercise and make more muscle, you will burn more calories when you are sleeping or sitting watching TV than you would have done without the exercise, and the new muscle.

Your body is adaptive and can run on a number of different fuels, with the exception of specialized parts such as your brain, which needs a constant supply of glucose. The body prefers to burn sugars, and the complex carbohydrates, which are long chains of sugars, are broken down to sugar to power the body and keep you alive.

LOW CARBOHYDRATE DIET

If there is no sugar available, your body will switch to burning fat. When you burn fat, you produce compounds called ketones, which can give your breath a sweet or sickly smell. They also tend to turn off your appetite and make it easier to reduce your food intake. This is the basis of a low carbohydrate diet, and why it is very effective at least in short-term weight loss. The concern here is that eating very few carbs leaves you predominantly eating animal products, and may dramatically increase your consumption of animal fats and cholesterol. The long-term implications of this are unclear. This diet, however, when it works, lowers the blood cholesterol level much more effectively than a diet that does not work and where the food is "healthy food" such as in the classical low-fat, high-fiber diet. The latter may contain a lot of carbohydrate, possibly explaining why it is often much less effective.

Remember your liver makes 80 percent of your cholesterol, and only a minority comes from your diet. It may not really matter how much you eat, your body just makes less to balance this.

There is no question fruit and vegetables are good for you in many ways. The problem comes in that some fruits and vegetables contain many carbohydrates, and in this type of diet, you need to carefully select them for low-carb content and take them in small amounts.

Ideally, a low-carb diet should include large amounts of fish and lean meat, unsweetened dairy products, small amounts of lower-carb fruit, vegetables, a fiber supplement, and supplementation with healthy oils rich in omega-3 fatty acids. Vitamin supplements may be helpful, and if continued long-term, consult a dietician or medical practitioner.

LOW–FAT, HEALTHY CARBOHYDRATE DIETS

Generally, a low-fat diet implies keeping dietary fat at less than 30 percent of the total calories, and healthy carbohydrates means fruit, vegetables, and grains. Add to this low-fat dairy, lean meat, poultry, and fish. There is no question this is a healthy diet, but it doesn't seem to work outside studies. Researchers conduct most studies under ideal, not real world, conditions where a patient is constantly followed up and the message reinforced to see they are behaving and following the diet. In the real world, we don't check up on patients all the time and, perhaps we seem to fail when simply instructing a patient and sending them on their way. Below is an example of this approach being ineffective in a large well-known trial.

Barbara Howard et al. Low-fat dietary pattern and weight change over 7 years: the Women's Health Initiative Dietary Modification Trial JAMA. 2006;295(1):39.

Unfortunately, diets, unless very strictly followed, are not effective on their own, presumably because of the body's own defense mechanisms, which serve to increase appetite. A review of five large studies of low-carbohydrate verses low-fat diets show that, generally, the low-carbohydrate diets are more effective at six months, but by one to two years, they are equally effective or ineffective in maintaining weight reduction.

Alain J. Nordmann. Effects of Low-Carbohydrate vs Low-Fat Diets on Weight Loss and Cardiovascular Risk Factors. Arch Intern Med. 2006;166:285-293

MEDITERRANEAN DIET

There is something in the Mediterranean diet that protects against cardiovascular disease and cancer related death despite a moderate consumption of saturated animal fats. This diet includes a moderate amount of olive oil (monounsaturated fat), high consumption of vegetables, fruits, legumes and grains, and moderate dairy intake predominantly in the form of cheese. This type of diet, if restricted, is similar in efficacy to those above with respect to weight loss and is also put forward by doctors and dieticians as a way of reducing heart and vascular disease in addition to weight loss.

Francesco Sofi et al. Adherence to Mediterranean diet and health status: meta-analysis. BMJ. 2008;337:a1344

The bottom line is weight loss is possible but does require lifestyle changes that include reduction in energy intake preferably combined with exercise, continued in the long-term. No one diet suits everyone; they work if you can stick to them, but this seems in reality to be rarely possible. Surgery is an effective alternative, especially in those in the higher weight range who have failed numerous attempts at weight loss with diet while awaiting a more effective medical therapy or magic pill.

"Diets don't work, I've tried them all!"

Is that so? Well, it was not the diet that failed; it was you, as hard as you no doubt find that to accept. Diets work, the problem is maintaining the new habits long-term. This is not rocket science, and I am sorry I do not believe there is a magical reason you regained your weight. What you need to do is look critically at what you are doing now (which is not working) and see where you can make changes.

Let's take sugar as an example. Apparently, thirty years ago the average sugar intake per person was about 3 kg per year in our society. Now it is more than 30 kg per year. Where is it? It is in almost all the processed foods you eat from bread buns, liquid sauces, fast foods, and especially in things you drink. What is the richest source of sugary drinks? Is it soft drinks or soda? No, it is actually the fruit juices in the non-refrigerated aisles in the supermarket. Those mixed juices are often 10 percent sugar by weight. That means 1 liter contains 100 g, which is about one-fifth of the height of the bottle, given sugar is much lighter than the water, but it is undetectable once dissolved in it.

The simple process of *actively* thinking about what you put in your mouth and cutting out sugar from your diet may be the only dietary change you need to make to lose all your excess body fat.

FRUIT AND VEGETABLES

These are the unsung heroes. Generally speaking they are far less energy dense than processed foods containing a lot of sugar and fats. Fruit and vegetables may be the healthiest part of the Mediterranean diet conveying its benefits.

Regular consumption of fresh fruits and vegetables is associated with a lower risk of cancer, heart disease, vascular disease, diabetes, high blood pressure, and stroke. Impressive stuff! This may be due to the phytochemicals and antioxidants including the polyphenols. Often these things give the color to the fruits and vegetables, so generally speaking, the more colorful the better for you. They also contain many potentially beneficial vitamins and minerals. The problem here lies in trying to sort out exactly what it is that is good for you, it would not be easy to do a study on one fruit or vegetable as many are eaten together and often combined with other healthy foods such as nuts and whole grains.

Jimaima Lako et al. Phytochemical flavonols, carotenoids and the antioxidant properties of a wide selectian of Fijian fruit, vegetables and other readily available foods. Food Chemistry Volume 101, Issue 4, 2007, Pages 1727-1741

The implication here is that regular intake of juices has been associated with an increased risk of diabetes, with implications possibly for the rest of the metabolic syndrome. Green leafy vegetables on the other hand are protective for diabetes.

Lydia Bazzano et al. Intake of Fruit, Vegetables, and Fruit Juices and Risk of Diabetes in Women. Diabetes Care July 2008 vol. 31 no. 7 1311-1317

RED MEAT OR WHITE MEAT?

People have long been concerned about red meat and health particularly in relation to cardiovascular disease and cancers. Red and processed meats are associated with modest increases in total mortality (risk of dying), cardiovascular mortality, and cancer mortality when compared to white meat. These results are from a prospective study over ten years of 70,000 men and women. The relative risk was 1.31 for total mortality, 1.22 for cancer mortality, and 1.27 for cardiovascular mortality. A high, white-meat diet was associated with a reduced overall mortality. If these figures are a little confusing, a 1.27 increased risk of cardiovascular mortality means a 27 percent increased risk of dying from cardiovascular disease.

Rashmi Sinha et al. High intakes of red or processed meat may increase mortality. Arch Intern Med. 2009;169:543-545, 562-571.

There are a number of observational studies that link a high intake of red meat to hormone receptor-positive breast cancer and this remains of concern; however, the finding has not been confirmed in all prospective studies.

E Cho et al. Red Meat Intake and Risk of Breast Cancer Among Premenopausal Women. Arch Intern Med. 2006;166:2253-2259

Some studies link red meat consumption to some types of lung cancer with a risk of 1.7 times non-red meat eaters, unrelated to smoking. These studies tend to combine red meat and processed meats.

Tram Lam et al. Intakes of Red Meat, Processed Meat, and Meat Mutagens Increase Lung Cancer Risk. Cancer Res 2009;69(3):932–9

WHAT SORT OF FAT OR OIL SHOULD I EAT? BUTTER VERSUS MARGARINE?

From an energy point of view, all fats are created equal. Oil and fat can be interchanged; however, generally speaking, you may think of fat as oil that is solid at room temperature. They are both fatty acids (FA).

There is no difference in the calories (energy) between olive oil, animal fat, or any other fat, they are all about nine calories per gram.

Where other health implications are concerned, however, there are probably great differences between different types of oil or fat.

This is a complicated area of nutrition and we are still trying to sort out the "evidence." If you are feeling tired I would skip this section, as it is likely to put you to sleep; however, if you are interested I will attempt to clarify it.

Without worrying too much about the detailed chemistry, fatty acids in your diet are generally classified into saturated (SFA), monounsaturated (MUFA) and polyunsaturated (PUFA).

In food processing you can take things one step further where vegetable oils are treated chemically or partially hydrogenated in food manufacturing to make them solid at room temperature. Manufacturers have done this for a century, as vegetable oils treated this way are cheaper than animal fats and have a longer shelf life. This chemical treatment alters the physical properties of the fatty acids making them solid by producing what we call "trans" double bonds on the opposite side of the fatty acid molecule. We have only recently come to appreciate that this physical change has biological effects as well. In other words, the trans-fatty acids (TFA) produced in this process may have significant health implications when consumed. People use them widely in cooking, baking, and frying foods. What do you think makes margarine solid?

Neither plants nor animals produce trans-fatty acids naturally, excepting small amounts produced by bacteria in mammal's intestines (sheep, cattle, and goats); however, the natural TFAs in these animal products are different and may not have adverse implications for health. The vast majority of TFA that you consume comes from food processing or manufacturing.

Trans-fatty acids have a number of possible biological implications:

1. Increased inflammation with potential effects on any inflammatory process in the body, such as vascular disease, asthma, or arthritis

2. Increase in the levels of bad cholesterol (LDL) with implications for cardiovascular disease

3. Damage to the lining of arteries (endothelium) with the potential for inducing blockage or reduced blood flow

4. Increased insulin resistance and diabetes (animal studies only at present)

5. Weight gain and obesity with a tendency to deposit the fat as visceral (bad) fat with implications for the metabolic syndrome

---

Teegala et al. Consumption and Health Effects of Trans Fatty Acids: A Review. JOURNAL OF AOAC INTERNATIONAL VOL. 92, NO. 5, 2009, 1250-57

Saturated fat (SFA) means there are no double bonds between the chain of carbon atoms that make up this fatty-acid molecule. In other words, the chain is fully saturated with hydrogen molecules; hence, the name saturated fatty acid. This tends to make the fatty acids solid at room temperature as they "stick together." Animal fats (cream, cheese, butter, lard, or ghee) and some vegetable fats (coconut, palm kernel, cotton seed, and chocolate) contain SFAs.

Monounsaturated fat (MUFA) means there is only a single double bond in the long carbon chain making up this fatty acid molecule. It is intermediated in physical properties being liquid at room temperature and solid in the fridge. Red meat, whole milk products, nuts, and high fat fruits such as olives and avocados contain MUFAs.

Polyunsaturated fat (PUFA) means there are multiple double bonds in the long carbon chain that makes up this fatty acid molecule. As the molecules do not stick together as well, they are generally liquid at room temperature and in the fridge. Nuts, seeds, fish, and green leafy vegetables contain PUFAs. This includes most vegetable oils you are familiar with. It may be in margarine but probably partly as hydrogenated TFAs to make it solid.

Do I really need to know all this?

Well I think you need to have some idea of what you are eating for the reasons to follow. It is also useful to be able to judge the fat simply by looking at it; if it is solid at room temperature, it is probably not good for you. Did you see what they fried your fish and chips in? It was very likely solid at room temperature, either SFA or TFA, both of which are bad for you. Don't let the sign "cooked in pure vegetable oil" mislead you. It was very likely TFA vegetable oil with significant health implications.

In a meta-analysis of nearly 350,000 people followed for up to 10 years, the risk of a dying from a heart attack was 26 percent lower if you swapped your intake of SFA for PUFA at a level of only 5 percent of your energy intake. If you did the same switching of SFA to carbohydrate, you actually increased your risk for a heart attack by 7 percent. Swapping SFA for MUFA in this study had no effect.

In other words, carbohydrate may be worse for you than saturated fat, and only a small change in the type of fat you consume may have a very significant effect on your risk for cardiovascular disease. PUFA (most vegetable oils) would seem to be the most protective here.

Patty Siri-Tarino et al. Meta-analysis of prospective cohort studies evaluating the association of saturated fat with cardiovascular disease. Am J Clin Nutr 2009;89:1425–32.

Dietary supplements

The reason that many dietary supplements are considered beneficial, at least in theory, is because they may have antioxidant properties. Antioxidants are chemical substances that gather up potentially damaging free radicals.

These free radicals are molecules that carry an extra electron or negative charge, which makes them very good at reacting with other molecules—such as the ones in your DNA—and consequently damaging them, sometimes irreparably. Various forms of radiation produce free radicals be it from the sun, a fluorescent light, or nuclear radiation. Free radicals are also produced by the simple process of consuming oxygen in chemical reactions in your body, which has to occur to keep you alive. We believe that if you have antioxidants present in your cells to mop up the free radicals, perhaps you will suffer less damage to your DNA, resulting in less disease and a longer life. There is probably some truth to this, and it may well explain the protective effect of fresh fruit and vegetables, which are loaded with antioxidants, as are many other food substances, such as coffee and chocolate (cocoa).

Unfortunately, nothing is ever as simple as it appears, and the implication that "if a little bit is good, more must be better" is not necessarily the case. This is especially true when using purified supplements such as vitamins, minerals, or chemicals with antioxidant properties.

Vitamins

Vitamins are essential nutrients. By this, we mean that the body cannot make them itself and has to get them from diet or other sources, such as sunlight (vitamin D).

VITAMIN A

Vitamin A is important for vision, especially at night, for bone growth, and for immune function. Animal products, dairy products, and colorful fruit and vegetables contain it. Excessive intake damages the liver, central nervous system, and bones, causing birth defects in unborn children and osteoporosis.

Vitamin A has long been known to possess antioxidant properties, so much so that millions of people have taken it as a supplement. The medical profession has trialed it to see if it can prevent cancer in some of those most at risk of this disease, such as lung cancer in cigarette smokers.

In one of the most famous studies looking at antioxidants, 18,314 smokers, former smokers, or those who had been exposed to asbestos were treated with vitamin A and beta carotene (an antioxidant plant pigment) or identical appearing placebo (sugar tablets). This was a group of people at high risk for developing lung cancer, and it was hoped the antioxidant combination would prevent at least some of the cancers.

What happened, to the investigators amazement, was unfortunately the reverse of this. After four years of treatment, the people taking the antioxidants were 1.5 times as likely to have died of lung cancer and 1.3 times more likely to have died from cardiovascular disease. As a result, they abandoned the study and stopped twenty-one months earlier than planned, as it appeared the active treatment group was suffering harm, not help, from the treatment.

Gilbert S et al. Effects of a Combination of Beta Carotene and Vitamin A on Lung Cancer and Cardiovascular Diisease. New Engl J Med,1996;334:1150-5.

I include this study to make the point that there is a lot we do *not* understand in this area of medicine, and just because it seems likely theoretically that something will do you good, in reality, this may not be the case at all. This is the point of an evidence-based approach to recommendations where possible. If something seems like a good idea and we feel it will do no harm, we subject it to rigorous testing in carefully conducted medical studies to attempt to prove our theories are correct before recommending it to the public. This is not always possible, and some of the recommendations in this book are yet to be formally tested in adequately sized, prospective randomized, double-blind studies, as was the example above. Remember, these type of studies are the highest quality evidence, as they move forward in time (prospective) and neither the investigators nor the patients know who is getting the active treatment (double-blind), reducing the risks of biased result.

We do not recommend taking this vitamin in large amounts, as it is likely to do more harm than good

VITAMIN D

Vitamin D is an extraordinary vitamin to say the least. The list of diseases that are more common in people with low vitamin D levels seem to increase on a daily basis. Beware this does not prove they are causatively associated. For example, patients with bowel cancer may have a low vitamin D level because they feel unwell and do not go outside in the sun (which raises vitamin D levels), rather than because the low vitamin D level increased the risk of cancer. I think there is reason for cautious optimism that raising the vitamin D levels in the community may reduce the burden of some diseases on society.

We believed until relatively recently that vitamin D was only associated with bone health and calcium absorption, preventing thin or weak bones. This is far from the truth, however, with many cell types throughout the body having receptors for this vitamin, indicating it has an effect on them.

The potential sites for action of vitamin D include but are not limited to:

Bone:

It is essential for the regulation of calcium absorption and bone strength. Deficiency causes "rickets" where bones have too little calcium and bend and break.

Cardiovascular disease:

It potentially prevents blockage of arteries in the heart and elsewhere by multiple actions, which include lowering blood pressure, reducing growth of smooth muscle in the walls of arteries, and reducing inflammation and calcification in the walls of arteries. All of which can lead to premature blockage. This may result in a heart attack or stroke as a result.

Immune function:

It stimulates immune function to fight infection by acting directly on several important immune-fighting cells (macrophages and neutrophils) leading to lower susceptibility to many infections including the flu, tuberculosis, and pneumonia.

It also seems to modulate the immune system to reduce the risk of autoimmune diseases, such as type 1 diabetes, rheumatoid arthritis, multiple sclerosis, and inflammatory bowel disease. Some studies show supplementation may reduce the development of some of these diseases.

Cancer:

Vitamin D has many effects in inhibiting cell growth, increasing cancer cell death (apoptosis), and inhibiting growth of blood vessels into cancer tissue. This reduces oxygen and nutrient supply and increases cell differentiation to stable mature noncancerous cells. Higher levels may reduce the risk of development and rate of growth of colon, pancreatic, breast, prostate, and ovarian cancers, as well as some lymphomas and melanoma. This is still unproven, however.

Muscle:

It increases muscle growth and strength—especially important in the elderly with increased risk for falls. It may also be important in maintaining healthy heart muscle.

Skin:

It improves skin health, with improvement in diseases, such as psoriasis.

Diabetes:

It possibly protects from both type 1 (childhood onset) and type 2 (obesity/exercise related) diabetes by modifying immune function, improving insulin sensitivity, and possibly stimulating insulin secretion.

So, how do you take vitamin D and how much is too much? Well, as we learn more about this vitamin we keep increasing what we feel is the minimal amount we should have in our blood stream. This was until recently 25 nmol/l and increased to 50, but should be 75–100 in my view, and the recommendations are likely to increase again.

Your skin produces the vitamin from cholesterol on exposure to UV light, and generally, ten to fifteen minutes in the sun per day will give you adequate levels; however, sun intensity is variable in different places and at different times of the day. Seek medical advice if going this route and remember the darker your skin the more sun exposure you will need. You can take it as a supplement called vitamin D3, which comes as 1000 IU in various forms. It is safe to take, and to ingest a toxic level (which is possible) you need very large amounts. A reasonable amount would be at least 1000 IU per day. A recent study comparing 3000 IU per day for three months followed by 1000 IU per day for two months, with 50,000 IU per day for ten days, were equally effective in treating deficiency with no toxicity in either group.

Medical Journal of Australia, Vol 192 Number 12, 21 June 2010

Remember, just because it sounds like "more must be better" on theoretical grounds, does not prove taking more will help more. Observational studies, where low levels appear to be associated with cancer, have suggested that antioxidants, such as beta-carotene, vitamin C, vitamin E, folic acid, and selenium should be good for you in higher doses. When subjected to more rigorous testing, however, in randomized controlled trials, they have not yet been shown to be of any benefit in reducing cancer risk, and some have even caused harm, as per the study example earlier of vitamin A.

Having given this warning, hopefully vitamin D will prove beneficial. As yet, no large-scale, randomized clinical trial of vitamin D supplementation and cancer risk as the primary endpoint has been done. Observational studies in breast cancer yield conflicting results. Similar studies in bowel cancer are generally promising with all suggesting protection or, at worst, no effect and no toxicity. Studies show conflicting results with uterine, esophageal, stomach, kidney, pancreatic, and ovarian cancer, and non-Hodgkin's lymphoma.

We desperately need some good quality, prospective, randomized-control studies to prove moderate to high-dose supplementation is beneficial before offering any black and white recommendations. At present, "the experts" would say there is evidence only for its use in protecting bones and muscle strength.

JoAnn Manson et al. Vitamin D and Prevention of Cancer – Ready for Prime Time? New England Journal of Medicine, Perspective, 1385-1387, 14 April 2011.

OTHER VITAMINS

As mentioned above, many vitamins have strong antioxidant properties, and it was hoped they would prevent diseases when used in higher doses, but as yet, this has not been proven.

They are still essential and here are the main associated deficiency syndromes:

Vitamin A	Dry eyes, blindness, dry skin
Vitamin D	Rickets
Vitamin E	Anemia
Vitamin K	Bleeding (failure of blood to clot)
Vitamin C	Scurvy, (fragile connective tissue and capillaries with easy bruising)
Vitamin B1 (Thiamine)	Nerve (neuropathy), heart (cardiomyopathy) and brain (encephalopathy) function problems
Vitamin B2 (Riboflavin)	Skin rash (dermatitis)
Niacin	Dermatitis, dementia, diarrhea
Vitamin B6 (Pyridoxine)	Inflamed tongue, neuropathy
Folate	Anemia
Vitamin B12 (Cobalamin)	Anemia, dementia, spinal degeneration

Minerals

There are numerous minerals that make up your body and many are essential for various body functions. For example, your blood could not carry oxygen without iron, and you could not stand up without calcium, as your bones would be like soft rubber. Your brain and heart could not function without sodium and potassium, which carry a charge and, therefore cause electrical activity when they move across cell membranes. This is essential to make your heartbeat or your brain think.

SODIUM (NA)

Mixed with chloride this makes common table salt. It is necessary for many functions but predominantly holds water in the blood stream and, thus, maintains blood volume. It keeps fluid in the extracellular space, outside cells, which includes the blood stream.

POTASSIUM (K)

This, again, has many functions including normal rhythm of the heart and muscle contractility, as well as being the main salt that keeps fluid inside cells, maintaining the intracellular space.

CALCIUM (CA)

Calcium has many functions in the body. Clearly one of the best known is the maintenance of strong and healthy bones. It stands to reason then that the more you take the stronger and healthier your bones will be, doesn't it?

Unfortunately, things are not that simple. If you simply take a lot of calcium as supplements, it does not necessarily go into your bones. Your body uses several mechanisms and hormones to carefully control the level of calcium in your blood, and high or low levels are toxic. If you take large doses of supplements, you will in the first instance get rid of the excess in your urine, which may put you at risk for kidney stones. You may also calcify soft tissues in your body, such as your blood vessels, thereby increasing your risk of vascular disease, such as heart attack and stroke.

A research paper in the British Medical Journal in 2010 reviewed fifteen studies looking at calcium supplementation of more than 500 mg daily and the risk of heart attack and stroke. The risk for heart attack was increased 1.3 times for those taking calcium compared to those taking placebo, and the risk of stroke showed a trend for an increased risk of 1.2 times.

Mark Bolland et al. Effect of calcium supplements on risk of myocardial infarction and cardiovascular events: meta-analysis. BMJ 2010;341:c3691

Does this mean that calcium in all forms is the same in increasing the risk of vascular disease? As you might expect, probably not is the answer. It may be safer to take calcium from food sources. A review of multiple studies of the intake of dairy products—the best source of dietary calcium—showed the reverse trend with respect to heart disease. The risk of heart attack was 0.87 for those taking higher levels of dairy foods, again stressing the point that it may be safer to take these things as whole foods not supplements.

Peter Elwood et al. The consumption of Milk and Dairy Foods and the Incidence of Vascular Disease and Diabetes: An Overview of the Evidence. Lipids (2010) 45:925–939

The implications from these studies are that taking large amounts of calcium supplements may be harmful, and you should avoid doing so.

Has your doctor advised you to take calcium supplements to prevent osteoporosis?

How much are you taking? Ask your doctor if it is OK for you to continue on this dose in light of recent studies.

IRON (FE)

Meat, fish, and chicken provide abundant amounts that can be easily absorbed. It is not really very bioavailable to the body (easily absorbed) from vegetable sources such as green leafy vegetables.

Iron is involved in many processes in the body. It enables your blood to carry oxygen around the body as it is an essential part of the protein haemoglobin, which performs this function.

Iron deficiency is common and it is caused by inadequate diet, poor absorption, or loss of iron due to loss of blood, for example, menstrual blood loss.

It is very toxic in large amounts and you should *only* take it as a supplement to treat deficiency states. Like most of these minerals, too much can kill you.

MAGNESIUM (MG)

Found in whole grains, legumes, and dark-green leafy vegetables

It is very important in cardiac and nervous function preventing disturbances in cardiac rhythm (arrhythmias) and in preventing excessive brain electrical activity disorders such fitting or seizures. It tends to calm down excitable components in the body. It also relaxes the muscle in blood vessels to lower blood pressure and in the airways to help prevent asthma. High compared to low intake seems to protect against diabetes and improves insulin sensitivity. Good stuff!

Taken orally in large amounts it acts as a laxative. It is relatively nontoxic; however, very large doses intravenously will stop your heart contracting and stop you breathing.

Trace Minerals

Trace minerals are, by definition, minerals you need in very small amounts; however, they are still important, and deficiency can cause severe disease or death. Generally speaking, they are also relatively toxic in large amounts with a very narrow "therapeutic window" being the range between deficiency and toxicity. This makes some of them relatively dangerous to take in significantly increased amounts. Deficiency states are uncommon in normal people and supplementation is not generally recommended. They include the following with the dietary sources listed.

CHROMIUM (CR)

Vegetables, grains, fruits

Deficiency is very rare outside hospitalized patients. Low levels may increase the likelihood of diabetes and possibly the metabolic syndrome. High levels of some forms may increase the likelihood of lung cancer. Body builders beware, there is no evidence it increases muscle mass as is a popular belief.

COPPER (CU)

Vegetables, meat

Yes, the same thing the water pipes in your house are made of but in another form as a "salt." It is very important. Deficiency can cause lack of skin pigmentation, muscle weakness, neurological problems, and weak bones. Excess causes liver failure and damage to the brain.

FLOURIDE (FL)

Water, seafood

Seems to have some beneficial effects in preventing dental caries and possibly in bone health; however, it is uncertain if this element is "essential" to us. Many water supplies add it for reduction of dental caries. Excessive intake leads to mottling of the teeth and to denser but weaker bones.

IODINE (I)

Salt, seafood, vegetables, drinking water

This is a very important element, and so much so that manufacturers add it to your diet in bread, salt, and water in many countries. It is important for normal functioning of your thyroid gland, and deficiency results in lower metabolic rate and intellectual impairment, often with a goitre or large thyroid gland visible in the neck. It is relatively nontoxic, except paradoxically in deficient states, where doctors need to administer it carefully.

MANGANESE (MN)

Meat, fish, poultry

Deficiency is not recognised in humans; in experimental animal studies, it can cause poor growth, bony disease, and abnormal metabolism.

Toxicity (welding and steel industries, water contamination) may cause brain and liver damage.

SELENIUM (SE)

Seafood, meat, grains

Selenium was another compound for which there was great optimism for preventing cancer. This was largely because low levels in the blood seemed to correlate with higher prevalence of some cancers and it functions in part as a strong antioxidant. Some studies show that supplementation in those with low levels reduces prostate cancer incidence.

Duffield-Lilico et al. Selenium supplementation, baseline plasma selenium status and incidence of prostate cancer: an analysis of the complete treatment period of the Nutritional Prevention of Cancer Trial. BJU International Volume 91, Issue 7, pages 608–612, May 2003

Studies have looked at selenium levels comparing high and low levels showing a 20 percent reduction in the chance of dying from all causes and a 30 percent reduction in the chance of dying from cancer with high levels; however, at very high levels the chance of dying from all causes begins to increase again.

Joachim Bleys et al. Serum Selenium Levels and All-Cause, Cancer, and cardiovascular Mortality Among US Adults. Arch Intern Med. 2008;168(4):404-410

Deficiency may result in skeletal and heart muscle problems, depression, and impaired immune function.

The early data for selenium was very promising; however, the problem with supplementation is the toxicity issue, and it does have a very narrow range of safety (therapeutic index). Excessive supplementation causes hair and nails to fall out, nervous system damage, and skin problems.

ZINC (ZN)

Animal products, nuts

Zinc is important for growth and tissue repair, sexual function, healthy skin, taste, smell, and immune function.

Severe zinc deficiency is uncommon in western society, as protein malnutrition is uncommon. It does correlate with markedly impaired immune function. In third world, where deficiency states are relatively common, there are numerous studies show zinc supplementation is effective in improving the outcome in severe diarrhoea and chest infection, particularly in children.

Bhutta et al. Therapeutic effects of oral zinc in acute and persistent diarrhoea in children in developing countries; Pooled analysis of randomized controlled trials. American Journal of Clinical Nutrition, Vol. 72, No. 6, 1516-1522, December 2000

It seems to work both to prevent the infections (even if given to pregnant women before children are born) and to treat them when they occur, possibly even when the child is not zinc deficient. It may shorten duration of the common cold and reduce the likelihood of dying from malaria.

So should we be taking it? Possibly, in modest amounts; however, it does interfere with the absorption of copper and may cause copper deficiency if taken in excess for long periods. Taking very large amounts will produce damage to the gut and cause kidney failure.

I make suggestions related to taking vitamins and mineral supplements later in this book.

Foods warranting special mention

CHOCOLATE

Chocolate is made from the cocoa bean, and in terms of health benefits, the darker the better. White or milk chocolate is essentially just fat and sugar mixed together with some flavoring, and it will do nothing other than help you put on weight.

Dark chocolate is something entirely different. Over the last fifteen years, numerous publications have shown benefit to health in consuming dark chocolate. Cocoa—the active ingredient—is rich in compounds called polyphenols, which are also present in red wine, green tea, and olive oil. They are powerful antioxidants. They, or something else in the cocoa, appear to have multiple health benefits including reduction of blood pressure, reduction in bad cholesterol (LDL), increase in good cholesterol (HDL) levels in the blood, improved insulin sensitivity (reduced diabetes), and in one study, it appeared to reduce the overall risk of dying, and dying from cardiovascular disease in elderly men. These comments are from a review of twenty-eight pub-lished studies in the literature, and many of the studies show the benefits.

Brian Bjijsse et al. Cocoa Intake, Blood Pressure, and Cardiovascular Mortality. Arch Intern Med 166, 411–417.

Karen Cooper et al. Cocoa and health: a decade of research. British Journal of Nutrition (2008), 99, 1–11

Chocolate contains numerous compounds that may offer health benefits. These include:

Theobromine, which is a stimulant similar to caffeine

Caffeine in small amounts

Tryptophan, which is an essential amino acid, increases the levels of serotonin in the brain. Serotonin reduces anxiety and is a centrally acting antidepressant.

Compounds that induce the release of endorphin-like sub-stances (natural opiates having effects like morphine or heroin), elevating mood and reducing pain.

Phenols are potent natural antioxidants. These potential-ly protect against cardiovascular disease and cancer. Chocolate is the highest known natural source of these substances. They are likely to be the cause of the dilation of blood vessels (reducing blood pressure), the documented changes in the good and bad cholesterol, and inhibition of platelet aggregation (blood clotting), which reduces the risk of vascular disease. The antioxidant effects reducing free radicals may reduce cancer incidence and protect against aging.

Anandamide, a compound that acts on the same receptors in the brain as marijuana, cause a feeling of well-being and reduced anxiety.

No wonder it makes you feel so good, it is like smoking a joint while injecting yourself with heroin and taking antidepressants by mouth all at the same time. And it is legal!

Potential disadvantages include effects on childhood hyperactivity, headache, heartburn induced by relaxation of the lower oesophageal sphincter by theobromine, allergic reactions, and weight gain depending on the form taken.

COFFEE

Coffee contains more than a thousand chemicals, many of which exert effects on those who drink it.

Caffeine is one of the best known of these and is a stimulant that increases mental alertness, raises blood pressure, increases metabolic rate, and causes a diuresis (increased urine production). Increasing your metabolic rate may help in weight loss, as you burn more calories, and the effect on metabolic rate lasts for twenty-four hours. (I hope you didn't put sugar in the coffee!)

There are other chemicals in coffee that may raise cholesterol, but this seems dependent on how a person brews it, and this does not translate into increased cardiovascular disease in larger studies.

The phenols in coffee are chlorogenic acids, and these are a potential source of its antioxidant activity. Other components include magnesium, potassium, niacin, and vitamin E, all of which may have health benefits but are present in small amounts only.

There is something in coffee that seems to protect you from developing *type 2 diabetes*, one of the major components of the metabolic syndrome. Most, but not all, studies (six of nine reviewed) show an inverse relationship between the amount of coffee intake and the risk of diabetes. In some studies, heavy drinkers reduced the risk by 50 percent or more (six cups per day). These were large prospective studies following groups (cohorts) of people up to 84,000 in size. The effect is dose dependent; the more you drink the less likely you are to get maturity onset diabetes.

Benjamin Schaefer. Coffee consumption and risk for type 2 diabetes mellitus. Ann. Intern. Med., 140:1–8.

The effect would appear to be very real. It is independent of caffeine with decaffeinated coffee showing the same effect. Tea by contrast in several large studies showed no effect. The effect is most likely to relate to the antioxidants (chlorogenic acid), but this is not really known.

There are also a number of large studies showing coffee and caffeine intake are inversely associated with the likelihood of developing *Parkinson's disease*, a degenerative neurological disease that often proves fatal over a number of years. In some studies, the effect seemed very powerful with a reduction in the likelihood of three to five times. Tea possibly works here too.

Ross et al. Association of coffee and caffeine intake with the risk of Parkinson disease. JAMA., 283:2674–2679.

Some researchers' associate coffee with a reduced risk of *suicide*, again in a dose-dependent fashion with a decreased risk of 13 percent per cup consumed daily in some studies or 50 percent reduction for at least two cups per day in other studies.

Kawachi et al. A prospective study of coffee drinking and suicide in women. Arch. Intern. Med., 156:521–525.

Arthur Klatsky et al. Coffee, tea, and mortality. Ann. Epidemiol., 3:375–381.

Coffee and the *liver*. Coffee's effect on the liver is nothing short of dramatic.

It appears to protect against inflammation in the liver and the end result of long-term inflammation, being cirrhosis and liver cancer.

It protects against liver toxins (poisons) such as alcohol, iron over load and fatty liver, as well as the effect of viruses (viral hepatitis).

Tommaso Stroffolini et al. Interaction of alcohol intake and cofactors on the risk of cirrhosis. Liver International Volume 30, Issue 6, pages 867–870, July 2010

The good news for alcohol drinkers is that coffee is effective at preventing damage to the liver with a linear reduction in the risk of developing cirrhosis of 22 percent per cup of coffee consumed. It also has a dose-dependent effect on reducing the acute effect of alcohol (alcoholic hepatitis) by about 20 percent per cup of coffee consumed daily, and up to 80 percent for four cups per day.

Coffee protects against fatty liver disease, and again, the more the better for this effect.

Does coffee consumption protect against cancer? The bottom line here is there does not appear to be any effect, either way. The earlier studies from twenty years ago suggesting a link were most likely confounded by the fact coffee drinkers were more likely to be smokers. In those studies it was the smoking not the coffee that was responsible for the apparent increased incidence of cancer. Multiple early studies suggested it reduced the risk of bowel cancer, but subsequent larger prospective studies suggest there is probably no effect.

The exception to this is liver cancer. There are numerous studies including larger prospective studies that show the more coffee you drink the less likely you are to get liver cancer. The commonest cause of cancer-related death on this planet is liver cancer, largely related to chronic hepatitis B and perhaps hepatitis C infection. The good news is it seems to work in these diseases with potentially great benefit worldwide.

Francesca Bravi et al. Coffee drinking and hepatocellular carcinoma risk: a meta-analysis. Hepatology Volume 46, Issue 2, pages 430–435, August 2007

GREEN TEA

"The experts" have considered green tea to possess various health promoting properties for centuries. It does indeed contain many polyphenols (antioxidants) that account for 30 percent of its dry weight, and it is these that may be responsible for health-promoting effects. At least in theory they may reduce the risk of cardiovascular disease, diabetes, and cancer, as well as having a potentially positive effects on inflammation, infections, and arthritis. A number of stud-ies show that when you look at populations drinking large amounts of green tea (five to six cups per day), they seem to have significantly less cardiovascular disease, lower blood pressure, lower incidence of stroke, lower cholesterol levels, less diabetes, and less likely to be obese, than comparison groups drinking small amounts (one cup or less). The trouble with this type of observational (epidemiological) study is what else do the groups do that is different from one an-other? Do those who drink tea drink less alcohol, for example? This is where it would be good if we had level-one evidence. However, these studies would be difficult to do because what would we use as the placebo?

In other words, it may be good for you, but we have not proven this yet. Some studies are in progress to give better levels of evidence, and I would be cautiously optimistic. In any case, it does not seem to do any harm, and if you are drinking it, don't stop, just continue, and wait for the evidence.

Swen Wolfram. Effects of Grean Tea and EGCG on Cardiovascular and Metabolic Health. Journal of the American College of Nutrition, Vol. 26, No. 4, 373S–388S (2007)

ALCOHOL AND RED WINE

Wine has been considered or perhaps hoped, by the healers of the day, to possess health benefits for thousands of years and was recommended for this reason by Hippocrates, the famous Greek physician, around 450 BC.

For several hundred years, doctors have noted that the French have a low incidence of heart disease despite a high intake of saturated animal fats. The medical profession has postulated this to relate to something in the Mediterranean diet. Red wine is a front-runner as the explanation.

Alcohol has been shown to give protection from heart disease, reducing the likelihood of heart attacks and reducing total mortality in numerous studies with a so-called J effect, where small doses are good but larger doses harmful. Regular moderate drinking raises the good cholesterol (HDL) and can increase insulin sensitivity reducing diabetes. Red wine alone potentially reduces the risk of ischemic stroke (from clots) whereas other alcohol has no effect. The risk of dying from heart disease is in several studies 25 to 50 percent lower in drinkers of one to three standard drinks per day than in nondrinkers.

Medical researchers feel this relates, in part at least, to the polyphenols in the red wine, especially resveratrol, which has numerous protective effects on the cardiovascular system. The actions of these polyphenols in red wine are similar to those in dark chocolate or cocoa. Red wine is the only type of alcohol where if your take the alcohol out, the remaining compounds appear to have protective benefits.

Corder et al. Redwine, chocolate and vascular health: developing the evidence base. Heart 2008;94:821-823 doi:10.1136/hrt.2008.143909

The news is not all good for alcohol. If you exceed two to three standard drinks per day your risk of dying from any cause increases again to become more than a non-drinker.

There is no J or U in the curve for the incidence of cancer. Any alcohol intake seems to increase the risk of cancer and this risk includes many common cancers, such as breast, bowel, throat, esophagus, and liver. It does not seem to matter what type of alcohol you drink, they all do it, and the more you drink the higher the risk. Presumably, you get a reduction in all-cause mortality with one to three drinks per day because the protective effect on cardiovascular disease outweighs the negative effect on cancers. The article below reviews the potential mechanisms for alcohol causing cancer.

Keith Singletary. Alcohol and Cancer; Biological basis. Nutrition and Health, 2010, Part 4, 735-760, DOI: 10.1007/978-1-60761-627-6_31

This effect is well quantified in studies involving bowel cancer, where anything over one drink per day can be shown to increase your risk.

Fedirko et al. Alcohol drinking and colorectal cancer risk: an overall and dose–response meta-analysis of published studies. Annals of Oncology Volume 22, Issue 9 Pp. 1958-1972

OLIVE OIL

Olive oil plays a large part in the Mediterranean diet and may make up 20 percent of the calories in this type of diet. It is difficult to separate the effects of the oil from the other components of the diet. Health care professionals have long suspected that it is the olive oil that conveys many of the health benefits, both on theoretical grounds and based on interventional studies. Adherence to a Mediterranean diet has been shown in studies to be associated with reduced overall mortality and longevity in Mediterranean and non-Mediterranean countries.

Pagona Lagiou et al. Mediterranean dietary pattern and mortality among young women: a cohort study in Sweden. Br J Nutr. 2006;96:384-92.

Antonia Trichopoulou et al. Modified Mediterranean diet and survival: EPIC-elderly prospective cohort study. BMJ. 2005;330:991-7

Some studies show olive oil itself lowers blood pressure and bad cholesterol and prolongs survival of diabetics.

A Trichopoulou et al. Olive oil, Mediterranean diet and health. J Intern Med. 2006;259:583-91.

It is not clear what it is in olive oil that conveys the benefits. Olive oil is high in monounsaturated fatty acids (a type of oil or fat), which may convey protective effects, especially on the cardiovascular system.

It also contains many other components, especially virgin olive oil. Many of these so-called minor components are polyphenols similar to those in red wine and cocoa, but unfortunately, up to 80 percent of these are lost in the refining process. Experimental studies show the compounds to be antioxidants, to protect the lining of blood vessels, to lower blood pressure, to prevent plate-let clumping (beginning of blood clotting process), and to pre-vent oxidation of LDL cholesterol (which reduces its deposition in the walls of arteries). These effects are potentially good for the heart and blood vessels. Animal models show them to delay progression of atherosclerosis (arterial disease).

The evidence for intervention causing benefit in humans is less impressive, but it is early days yet. Laboratory based studies have shown it to have an antioxidant effect in the blood, and virgin olive oil particularly is associated with lower blood pressure and reduction in the need for blood-pressure medication. The fact that this effect predominantly relates to virgin olive oil suggests it is the minor components, such as the polyphenols, not the type of oil, that convey the benefits.

L. Aldo Ferrara et al. Olive Oil and Reduced Need for Antihypertensive Medications Arch Intern Med. 2000;160:837–842.

Eric L. Ding et al. Optimal Dietary Habits for the Prevention of Stroke Am J Clin Nutr. 2004;80:1012–1018.

Remember, a lot of the evidence cited here comes from basic research (in the laboratory) and observational studies of populations. The level-one (best) evidence we require to make dietary recommendations (randomized, double-blind, prospective studies) is still in the pipeline, outcome uncertain.

FISH OIL

Fish oil is rich in a particular type of fat called omega-3 fatty acid. Epidemiological studies from up to forty years ago have suggested a link between high intake of these fatty acids and reduced cardiovascular death, and these findings have been confirmed in subsequent higher quality interventional studies in both disease prevention (primary prevention) and treatment after an event (secondary prevention).

This effect is confined to the true cold-water fish oils (eicosapentaeonic or EPA and docosahexaenoic or DHA as opposed to a similar plant derived omega-3 fatty acid called alpha-linolenic acid or ALA). The fish oil comes all the way up the food chain from the tiny phytoplankton in the sea. I give you the complicated names only so you can check your oil capsules and make sure you are not taking the plant extract, as this has not been shown to give protection. Only fish can turn it into fish oil, and humans convert less than 5 percent to the beneficial products (EPA and DHA).

An evidence based review of randomized controlled trials and observational studies published by Wang et al. in 2006 concluded:

"Most trials reported that fish oil significantly reduced all-cause mortality, myocardial infarction (heart attack), cardiac and sudden death or stroke." Not all studies showed evidence for stroke reduction. The effect was greater for secondary than primary prevention; in other words, after a heart attack it prevented another one. The evidence was taken from forty-six separate studies analyzed and was only for EPA/DHA and not the plant derived ALA, which was not shown to be protective.

Richard J Deckelbaum et al. n–3 Fatty acids and cardiovascular disease: navigating toward recommendations. .Am J Clin Nutr 2006;84:5–17.

Fish oil may have a protective effect in a number of cancers including common western cancers, such as lung, breast, and bowel.

Theoretical reasons and laboratory-based experiments suggest fish oil may be useful to prevent or treat cancer.

A twenty-two year prospective study suggested a decreased risk of developing colorectal (bowel) cancer.

Megan N. Hall et al. A 22-year Prospective Study of Fish, n-3 Fatty Acid Intake, and Colorectal Cancer Risk in Men. Cancer Epidemiol Biomarkers Prev May 2008 17; 1136

Fish oil may be preventative in breast cancer, and current use has been associated with a reduced risk of developing breast cancer (by 30 percent), but this remains to be proven in high-quality studies.

Theodore M. Brasky et al. Specialty Supplements and Breast Cancer Risk in the VITamins And Lifestyle (VITAL) Cohort. Cancer Epidemiol Biomarkers Prev; 19(7); 1696–708. ©2010 AACR.

The bottom line here is we do not yet recommend this for cancer prevention or treatment, but it has very few side effects, perhaps apart from reflux and bad breath. It probably does protect you from heart disease.

TREE NUTS AND PEANUTS

Nuts have been part of the human diet for thousands of years and there is good epidemiological evidence for a protective effect on cardiovascular disease. An analysis of four large epidemiological studies suggests high nut consumption reduces your risk for dying from heart disease by about 35 percent.

There may be many reasons for this. Studies have shown a diet containing nuts to lower the bad cholesterol (LDL), to have anti-oxidant effects, to reduce inflammation, and to protect the lining of blood vessels (endothelium) from injury, thereby, potentially reducing the risk of clots and the buildup of plaque, which may narrow the arteries.

Nuts contain many nutrients that are presumably responsible for this, including monounsaturated fatty acids, polyphenols (antioxidants), and other bioactive compounds. As with many of the dietary components already mentioned, if we could increase the consumption of these across a community, this may result in significant reduction in heart disease.

Janet C. King et al. Second International Nuts and Health Symposium, 2007. J. Nutr. September 1, 2008 vol. 138 no. 9 1734S-1735S

SALT

Sodium chloride, sea salt, or table salt has long been considered a bad part of our diet. It is, however, essential for life; without it, we would die. The real question is how much do we need.

The medical profession credit salt as a major factor in increasing blood pressure—including in children—and consequently our risk for stroke and cardiovascular disease. At present about 25 percent of the adult population suffer from high blood pressure with enormous consequences for the health system. Any small change at a population level is likely to save billions in health care costs.

Having said this not everyone with high blood pressure is "salt sensitive." This applies to only 50 percent of patients with high blood pressure under forty years of age, with the percentage gradually increasing with age, to as much as 80 percent at age sixty. This seems to have something to do with the kidneys' ability to get rid of the salt, resulting in an increase in blood volume and consequently higher blood pressure, as you have a relatively fixed storage compartment for your blood. The detailed mechanism is not well understood by doctors and is still under research.

Martha Franco et al. Pathophysiology of Salt-Sensitive Hypertension: A New Scope of an Old Problem. Blood Purif 2008;26:45–48

A high salt intake has also been linked in the medical literature to a higher risk for stomach cancer, heart failure, and kidney failure.

In most cases, the food industry adds salt to your food and it's in sauces and the cooking process, at home or in a food manufacturers factory. The implication here is that taking the saltshaker off the dining table is not going to help much. A person would need to tackle the food manufacturers at a government level. The experts in this field of medicine postulate that doing so at this level and legislating for reduced salt levels in food would have very large positive effects on the health of the population in general, even though not everyone is "salt-sensitive."

The trouble is salt makes food taste better! Your taste buds require some salt to function optimally and this conditions us to enjoy a relatively high-salt diet.

Naturopathic medication/supplements

I will not review this topic in detail at this time for several reasons. These do *not* include my lack of belief in any natural medication having any benefit. Note all the natural foods and supplements already mentioned in the text and the evidence for benefits. Unlike many of my naturopathic colleagues, I do not believe "because it is natural it must be good for you." Does this include scorpion venom, for example?

The reasons for not going into detail here are firstly that this is not my area of expertise. I have spent the last thirty-four years studying medicine, patients, and medical diseases but not naturopathic medications. Bear in mind that many of our conventional medicines, from penicillin to heart drugs, do come from natural beginnings and many more will in the future.

The second reason for not reviewing the evidence for the efficacy of this type of medication is that there simply is very little good-quality evidence in the literature to review.

The medical profession, where possible, tests drugs and therapies rigorously to confirm they do no harm and do actually work before they recommend them. Unfortunately, the "natural healers" do not tend to do so, relying on faith, the placebo effect, and word of mouth passed down over generations.

So, while I firmly believe there is a lot out there with very real potential benefit to patients, I don't know what to recommend in an "evidence-free zone." The sooner we can begin testing many of these compounds the better for all concerned, particularly the patient.

I am not going to recommend something that no one has proven safe or beneficial, with the same standards of evidence discussed earlier in the book.

Conventional medications that may prolong life

ASPIRIN

Like many drugs, aspirin has many effects. These effects include anti-inflammatory, such as treating an inflamed joint, analgesic (pain relief) for headache or other pain, blood thinning (by inhibit-ing aggregation of platelets, which reduces clotting), and possibly cancer prevention to mention a few. Humans have used this relatively simple compound for more than a hundred years. Its drawbacks include the risk of stomach ulcers and increased risk of bleeding because of reduced blood clotting.

The medical profession has used aspirin for years mainly for prevention of cardiovascular disease in people who have had an event such as a stroke or a heart attack, in an attempt to prevent a recurrence. This is so-called "secondary prevention."

Numerous medical studies show aspirin for secondary prevention works well, preventing recurrent strokes or heart attacks and, unless there is a good contraindication, we use it widely in this situation.

An expert task force in the US recently reviewed published data to use aspirin for primary prevention (before anything has occurred). Their conclusions, bearing in mind there is not a lot of published literature, was that aspirin does prevent heart attacks in men and strokes in women. It did not seem to affect all-cause mortality for the duration of the studies looked at. The protection from ischemic strokes in men (because of blood clots) was balanced with an increased risk of hemorrhagic strokes (bleeding from burst blood vessels). There was an increased risk of bleeding from the gut in men and women.

Tracy Wolff et al. Aspirin for the Primary Prevention of Cardiovascular Events: An Update of the Evidence for the U.S. Preventive Services Task Force Annals of Internal Medicine, March 17, 2009 vol. 150 no. 6 405-410

More interesting is the effect of aspirin on cancer both in terms of reducing new cases and possibly in prolonging survival in patients who already have a diagnosis of cancer. This may relate to aspirin's effect on the chemicals in the body called prostaglandins, of which it inhibits the production. Prostaglandins have effects on tumor cell growth, tumor cell death (apoptosis), and the growth of blood vessels into the tumor to supply it with oxygen and nutrients for growth.

In western societies, the common causes of cancer death are lung, colorectal, breast, and prostate cancers, and aspirin seems to work to reduce these, as well as pancreas, stomach, and esophageal cancer.

J Cuzick et al. Aspirin and non-steroidal anti-inflammatory drugs for cancer prevention: an international consensus statement. The Lancet Oncology, Volume 10, Issue 5, Pages 501 - 507, May 2009

The risk reduction in colorectal (bowel) cancer, one of the biggest killers in our society and one of the best studied, is in the region of 30 to 70 percent reduction in regular aspirin takers. The risk reduction seemed to be greater for those who took larger doses, with 70 percent reduction at 600 mg per day. The effect takes about six years of continuous use before any benefit shows. Aspirin appears to reduce the chance of dying from bowel cancer after treatment, in other words, to reduce the risk of recurrence after the initial tumor has been surgically removed.

Andrew T. Chan et al. Aspirin Use and Survival After Diagnosis of Colorectal Cancer. JAMA. 2009;302(6):649-658.,

Andrew T Chan et al. Aspirin Dose and Duration of Use and Risk of Colorectal Cancer in Men. Gastroenterology Volume 134, Issue 1 , Pages 21-28, January 2008

Breast cancer is obviously a very common cancer in women but does occur in men. Aspirin is not clearly useful in preventing primary breast cancer but does seem to have a very significant effect on the likelihood of recurrence and death from secondary breast cancer, after treatment of the primary cancer.

Heather Eliassen et al. Use of Aspirin, Other Nonsteroidal Anti-inflammatory Drugs, and Acetaminophen and Risk of Breast Cancer Among Premenopausal Women in the Nurses' Health Study II. Archives of Internal Medicine 2009 Vol. 169 No. 2 pp. 115-121

Michelle D. Holmes et al. Aspirin Intake and Survival After Breast Cancer. American Society of Clinical Oncology, JCO March 20, 2010 vol. 28 no. 9 1467-1472

Overall, regular aspirin use clearly reduces the risk of cancer re-lated death, but probably only by about 10 percent.

L H Opie. Aspirin in the prevention of cancer. The Lancet, Volume 377, Issue 9759, Pages 31 - 41, 1 January 2011

If you are going to take it regularly, especially at the higher doses, you should discuss it with your doctor and consider tak-ing another medication to prevent it causing stomach ulcers.

People still die with bleeding ulcers, I should know, as I often have to get up in the middle of the night to treat these patients.

BLOOD PRESSURE MEDICATION (ANTIHYPERTENSIVES)

Blood pressure refers to the pressure within your arteries.

Within reason, the lower your blood pressure is the better, as long as this does not include you passing out or fainting on standing. Low blood pressure is certainly better than normal blood pressure with respect to the risk of cardiovascular disease, such as strokes and heart attacks. The higher your blood pressure the more likely these things are to occur.

There is no question if you have significantly raised blood pressure your medical practitioner will suggest you take antihypertensive medication to reduce your risk of the adverse events described above.

The question then arises, Should you be taking medication to get your blood pressure as low as possible within the normal/low range? I will return to this point; however, treatment, at least in theory, will reduce your risk of cardiovascular disease. The problem with this though is the potential side effects and the cost of the medication. The side effects are sometimes significant, and if there is only likely to be a small reduction in your risk for cardiovascular disease, medication may cause more trouble than it cures. Exercise, reduced dietary salt intake, and weight loss, which lower blood pressure effectively in most people, would surely be the best initial approach.

A recently published Italian study of nearly 19,000 newly diagnosed hypertensive (high blood pressure) patients beginning medication showed that at least 50 percent of patients treated did not adhere strictly to their medication, and only those who did adhere had a significant reduction in cardiovascular events such as heart attack or stroke (reduced by 38 percent). This is not 100 percent because age, obesity, diabetes, high cholesterol, and numerous other issues contribute to your risk for these diseases, independently of blood pressure.

Giampiero Mazzaglia. Adherence to Antihypertensive Medications and Cardiovascular Morbidity Among Newly Diagnosed Hypertensive Patients. Circulation. 2009;120:1598-1605.

Studies show that for patients without high blood pressure but with cardiovascular disease, treatment with antihypertensive therapy, to lower their blood pressure, does reduce future risk.

Statistically significant decreases in stroke (down 23 percent) heart attack (down 20 percent), heart failure (down 29 percent), and death (down 13 percent) have been demonstrated; however, you need to treat a moderate number of patients to prevent one event over five years of follow up. These are relatively recent figures from a review (meta-analysis) of twenty-five studies, and doctors are still discussing how to interpret this information.

AM Thompson et al. Antihypertensive Treatment and Secondary Prevention of Cardiovascular Disease Events Among Persons Without Hypertension. JAMA. 2011;305(9):913-922.

Now, what has all this got to do with you? Well, I'm afraid it gets even more complicated. The fact is that not all blood pressure tablets are created equal.

There is a very important system built into your body to help maintain your blood pressure, preventing it from going too low.

It comes into play particularly when you are dehydrated or salt deficient.

The problem here is that our current lifestyle seems to upset this, and as a result, it works too well. In an "exercise deficiency state," (did someone mention the metabolic syndrome?) this system seems to go haywire.

This system is called the renin-angiotensin-aldosterone-system (RAAS). It has the potential to damage your blood vessels, your kidneys, and your heart. Drugs that block this system have similarly large names including angiotensin-converting enzyme (ACE) inhibitors and angiotensin receptor blockers (ARB). These drugs, especially the ACE inhibitors are very effective in managing high blood pressure, diabetes, heart failure, cardiovascular disease, and kidney disease.

Heard of these diseases before? Yes, that's right; they are very much overrepresented in the metabolic syndrome.

The implication here is if you have risk factors for the metabolic syndrome, you could make a good argument for beginning treatment with an ACE inhibitor even if you do *not* have high blood pressure. I consider this second-line treatment, and I am assuming you have failed miserably in the first-line exercise, salt restriction, and weight loss arena.

The billion-dollar question again is, should "normal' people take ACE inhibitors or ARBs, and would they live longer and healthier lives? We don't know, but I suspect the answer may well be yes.

Why you say?

Well, I suspect for at least two reasons.

These drugs are effective in treating "hypertension" by which most doctors mean a blood pressure of greater than 140 mm Hg. Studies show, however, that taking the blood pressure down to 115 mm Hg and possibly lower, protects you from bad events like strokes and heart attacks. In other words, your doctor's definition of high blood pressure is probably wrong, and in an ideal world, we should be aiming for lower levels. As soon as you go over 115 mm Hg in blood pressure your risk for stroke and heart attack increases and perhaps this level, and not 140 mm Hg, should be where we discuss beginning therapy.

The second issue relates to dying of "natural causes." As I have mentioned before, there is no such thing!

What is the most common cause of death in the western world? Could it be cardiovascular disease? What is one of the most effective drugs we have for preventing cardiovascular and other diseases? That's right—it is an ACE inhibitor.

What does the literature say on this question, to treat or not to treat normal levels of blood pressure? Well, unfortunately, I am not aware of any studies as yet to quote and give you the evidence.

Do you remember what I said about expert opinion? Well I am afraid that includes me. When discussing treating people with normal blood pressure we are talking about level-four evidence. Do I take this medication? Yes, I do (when I remember), and I do not have high blood pressure or other risk factors.

CHOLESTEROL LOWERING MEDICATION (THE "STATINS")

If I have you confused about whether or not you should take blood pressure medication, things are only going to get worse.

These cholesterol lowering drugs do seem to have numerous potentially beneficial effects on a number of diseases; however, their use comes at a cost in terms of side effects as well as dollars.

High cholesterol is a risk factor for cardiovascular disease, and drugs that lower this should be beneficial. The pharmaceutical industry developed these drugs and they are very effective in lowering cholesterol because they inhibit your liver's ability to manufacture cholesterol. Most of the cholesterol (80 percent) comes from production within your body, not as many believe from eating too many eggs or too much cream.

Statins lower the bad cholesterol (LDL), slightly increase the good cholesterol (HDL), and lower the other bad fats called triglycerides. The latter are significantly raised in the metabolic syndrome.

The statin drugs have numerous effects not related to their cholesterol-lowering ability. These include anti-inflammatory, vascular, and immune-altering effects. Doctors prescribe these primarily for their effect on cardiovascular disease however. In the setting of cardiovascular disease, they significantly reduce the risk of a new event such as a heart attack if you have already suffered one, so-called secondary prevention. They also work in primary prevention if you have risk factors for a heart attack or stroke (did someone mention the metabolic syndrome again?) but do not have any established underlying cardiovascular disease.

For example, in someone who has uncomplicated high blood pressure and diabetes. In this setting, they reduce the risk of a heart attack by 30 percent, a stroke by 20 percent, and all-cause mortality (risk of dying) by 12 percent. This data is from ten trials involving more than 70,000 people.

J J Brugts et al. The benefits of statins in people without established cardiovascular disease but with cardiovascular risk factors: meta-analysis of randomised controlled trials. BMJ. 2009; 338: b2376.

Other possible positive statin effects:

Protection from dementia

C Cramer et al. Use of statins and incidence of dementia and cognitive impairment without dementia in a cohort study. Neurology July 29, 2008 vol. 71 no. 5 344-350

Protection from all cancer incidence 25 percent

Wildon Farwell et al. The Association Between Statins and Cancer Incidence in a Veterans Population. JNCI J Natl Cancer Inst (2008) 100 (2): 134-139.

Protection from prostate cancer, the latter reduced by 31 percent in statin takers in the following study

Wildon Farwell et al. Statins and Prostate Cancer Diagnosis and Grade in a Veterans Population. JNCI J Natl Cancer Inst Volume103, Issue11 Pp. 885-892.

Slightly reduced incidence of large bowel and rectal cancer

Marc Bardou et al. Effect of statin therapy on colorectal cancer. Gut 2010;59:1572-1585

Inhibition of breast cancer cell growth and recurrence

Michael Campbell et al. Breast Cancer Growth Prevention by Statins. Cancer Res September 1, 2006 66; 8707

The above cancer examples are for common cancers, and they may inhibit the growth of many other cancer cells.

Possible negative statin effects or side effects:

Slight increase in the risk of diabetes

Liver inflammation (rare)

Muscle inflammation, very common at a low degree, rarely severe; however, everyone taking these drugs develops changes in muscle on electron (very powerful magnification) microscopic examination of their muscle. The significance of this is uncertain.

The possibility of memory impairment.

Cost is always going to be an argument. Who is going to pay?

I have given you a lot of detail here on the statins because they are very effective drugs, and the question arises, should we all be taking them? Should people over fifty all be taking them? We do not know the answer to these questions, and clearly, they depend on a balance of positive versus negative effects including cost.

When prevention fails:
Screening for early cancer, does it help?

Cancer is a scary word for most of us. This is, I think, primarily because of the perception that the medical profession cannot cure it and it is essentially a death sentence. Unfortunately, this is often the reality. With all our best medical therapy in the twenty-first century, involving chemotherapy, radiotherapy, and surgery, many patients still fall through the net.

Every cell in your body that divides has the potential to lose the controlling mechanisms for cell division and cell death (apoptosis). The result is cancer, that has the ability to spread around the body and to stimulate blood vessels to grow into the new tumor to sustain it. You may be surprised to learn that most cancer deaths in this world relate to infections. The commonest cause of cancer related death worldwide is liver cancer or hepatoma. This results most often from chronic (long-term) hepatitis B virus infection causing inflammation in the liver. The second commonest cause worldwide is stomach cancer, which is the result of a chronic bacterial infection in the stomach called helicobacter pylori. People pick up both these infections in early childhood and they stay with them for life in one form or another.

So, how do you cure these cancers?

We stop people getting the infections in the first place by vaccination and public health measures or we treat them as soon as possible if people do contract infection. This has potentially huge ramifications for cancer related deaths, particularly in the developing world where these cancers are very common.

In the developed world, where most of the readers of this book live, things are a little bit different. Vaccination has taken care of hepatitis B infection, and sanitation (sewage systems) has taken care of helicobacter pylori. Consequently, liver and stomach cancers are much less common but do still occur.

LUNG CANCER

In our society, lung cancer is the most common form of cancer-related death in adults, and this is falling in incidence (but rising in the developing world). How do you avoid lung cancer? Well, that is a no brainer if ever there was one: you stop smoking. It will still occur if everyone stops smoking but would probably reduce by 90 percent with some still occurring by chance, air pollution in cities, asbestos exposure, or other mechanisms.

BOWEL CANCER

If you are a non-smoking person—taking men and women together—the second most common cause of cancer related death in our society is bowel (colon and rectum) cancer. As already discussed, the metabolic syndrome and perhaps red meat significantly increase the risk of this cancer. Aspirin and a high intake of fresh fruit and vegetables reduce it.

Even if you do everything right, you are still at risk. The lining of the bowel is under considerable stress in its normal function and the body replaces it frequently. This is in stark contrast to your brain cells, which are under no significant stress (particularly if you fail to heed the messages in this book) and do not divide in adulthood. Every division of cells in the bowel to make new cells is associated with the risk of errors in the DNA. To make matters worse, the cells in the bowel wall are in very close proximity to bacteria in the bowel lumen and these bacteria produce toxins that damage the dividing DNA, making those errors more common.

So, this is where screening comes in. If you cannot prevent the cancer in the first place, the best hope for curing a cancer is finding it early, before it spreads to areas where we cannot reach it. Every cancer, in theory at least, begins as one cell and then doubles relentlessly in cell numbers until it overcomes you. Screening means finding a cancer (or precancerous lesion) *before* you have any symptoms to suggest its presence. This makes a big difference to the outcome. For bowel cancer, for example, if you have symptoms at the time of diagnosis (bleeding, change in bowel habit, or pain), there is about a 50 percent chance you will be dead from it in five years even with everything modern medicine has to throw at you. If doctors find it on screening, the chance of dying from it within five years is only about 10 percent. To a lesser or greater extent this is true for most other cancers.

I am only going to cover common cancers, and I make no apologies for beginning with bowel cancer because, as mentioned, it is at the top of the pops, assuming no suicidal intent with cigarettes is at play. By the way, smoking increases the risk of most cancers including bowel, not just lung cancer.

In a way, we are very lucky with bowel cancer in that it begins with polyps. These are "pre-cancerous" or benign growths in the bowel that become cancers if you leave them long enough. The process of growing a polyp and it turning into a cancer may leave you a window of opportunity of five to ten years. Cutting them out during this time cures you of that particular bowel cancer, which was to occur at the site of the polyp, assuming you were not planning to die from something else in the meantime.

Now, there are a number of ways to screen for bowel cancer. You may like to have a simple blood test; however, once the available blood tests are positive, it is usually too late. We use these tests to look for recurrent disease after a person has had a bowel cancer surgically removed.

The simplest screening test is to test the bowel motions for blood; this is called fecal occult blood testing. Three large, prospective studies in the 1990s have been published showing a reduction in the chance of dying from bowel cancer in the region of 15 to 20 percent if you do the screening every one to two years. What happens if you do it every five to ten years? Well, no one knows, this is a *completely* evidence-free zone, which the Australian government currently funds to keep the ignorant voters quiet. Presumably, it will reduce mortality by a smaller amount than 15–20 percent, perhaps 10 percent or less. If you live in Australia this is what you have available.

Another modality often combined with fecal occult blood testing is flexible sigmoidoscopy. With flexible sigmoidoscopy, the doctor uses an endoscope to examine the left side of your large bowel. Studies suggest this reduces your risk of dying from bowel cancer by about 35 percent. The problem with flexible sigmoidoscopy is it looks at the left half of your bowel only, and does not usually get very good views, as the preparation of the bowel is often suboptimal. You would be correct in your assumption that looking at the left side of the bowel is better than no screening at all; however, half the cancers occur in the right side of the bowel. If you were a woman undergoing screening for breast cancer would you think it was reasonable to screen your left breast only?

I am going through this in some detail, as *your* doctor is going to suggest these screening modalities to you and I want you to be able to make an *informed* and *evidence-based* assessment. I have not given references for my figures here, as this is my area of specialty, and I know there are numerous studies to back up these figures.

So, what should you do to avoid dying from bowel cancer?

Colonoscopy is the current answer. The Governments of the United States and multiple European countries recommend this from about the age of fifty because they have read or been advised on the evidence.

Overall, colonoscopy reduces bowel cancer death rates by about 80 percent if you had one performed in the last ten years.

Hermann Brenner et al. Protection From Colorectal Cancer After Colonoscopy: A Population-Based, Case–Control Study. Annals of Internal Medicine, 2011;154:22-30

Colonoscopy involves examination of the whole colon after a patient has cleaned it out with oral preparation so we can see the polyps and cut them out. The drawbacks are expense and needing a whole day for the preparation of the bowel. You do not necessarily need sedation if you choose a reasonably skillful colonoscopist, as it is not particularly uncomfortable and takes about fifteen minutes. This also assumes you have a relatively normal bowel without any major hurdles for the colonoscopist.

I have had two without sedation, as have many of my colleagues. They are no big deal.

So, when your doctor says to you; "Let's discuss bowel cancer screening," your response should be, "what would you do?" I have not met a medical practitioner over fifty who would follow the Australian guidelines for bowel cancer screening, and have fecal occult blood testing. The "informed" medical practitioners know the results; they all have a colonoscopy.

BREAST CANCER

Now, if you happen to be a non-smoking woman, breast cancer is your commonest cause of cancer related death in the developed world. Your lifetime risk is about one in eight if you are born in the United States and is higher if you have a family history, as is the case with bowel cancer. Unfortunately, unlike bowel cancer, we are not able to detect any precancerous lesions, which become breast cancer, giving us a much smaller window of opportunity to make the diagnosis before it is too late. Unfortunately, we also do not have as good a tool to look for the early cancers and need to rely on x-rays of the breasts, so-called mammography. This test is of most use in women over fifty because in younger women, the breast is relatively dense and it is harder to see the new growths. Between the ages of forty and forty-nine there is not a clear consensus amongst experts as to the benefit of screening, and over age seventy, most do not recommend screening.

The concern about waiting is that once you can feel the tumor as a lump it may have already spread and be incurable.

Mammography purportedly reduces the risk of dying from breast cancer by about 25 percent (women aged fifty to sixty-nine years) and on this basis is what the World Health Organization recommends. This recommendation is based on at least three large randomized trials.

Nystrom L et al. Breast cancer screening with mammography: overview of Swedish randomised trials.

Lancet 1993;341:973-8

There is still a lot of argument about how effective the screening really is, however. At least half and perhaps two-thirds of the reduction may be simply because the screened women are much more aware of the disease and tend to regularly and carefully examine themselves. Added to this we are getting better at treating breast cancer, and the risk of dying if you have the disease was falling overall during the time of the study, meaning the screening itself may not have been the reason for the reduced mortality. A more recent review of the data from more than 40,000 women with breast cancer suggested that the real reduction in mortality (chance of dying) from breast cancer attributable to the screening with mammograms was closer to 10 percent or less, which is unfortunately relatively poor. We clearly need much better ways to screen for breast cancer. Added to this issue is the fact that x-rays can actually cause cancer, and it's possible the screening itself slightly increases the risk.

Kalager M et al. Screening vs Better Treatment: Which Is More Effective in Reducing Breast Cancer Mortality? N Engl J Med 2010;363:1203-10.,

PROSTATE CANCER

Now, when it comes to cancers only men have to worry about, things get even more dismal when discussing prostate cancer. The prostate gland is unfortunately stuck in a relatively inaccessible place, just under the bladder. You can really only reach it to examine it by putting a finger in the rectum—*ouch*! As you can imagine, many men are not particularly compliant in having this examined, as I am often told, "Stay away! That is a one way valve only!"

The bad news about prostate cancer is that it is very common, and if you are male and live long enough, you have a high risk of getting it. This makes it the commonest form of cancer in males. The good news is that it is a disease predominantly of older men, and it is unlikely to kill you, partly because it is often slow growing and partly because you are at high risk of dying from something else at that age!

Screening for prostate cancer takes two main forms. One is a blood test called prostate specific antigen (PSA) and the other is the "finger" (hopefully gloved), the so-called digital rectal examination (DRE).

There is a lot of ongoing argument about screening for prostate cancer for two reasons.

One is that it may not work, or in other words, does not reduce the risk for death from the disease. A recent comprehensive review of DRE and PSA together done in a group of 76,693 men, randomised to screening or no screening, with follow up for seven to ten years. The screening in this study had no influence on death from prostate cancer. The compliance with screening was about 85 percent, which is relatively good.

Fritz H. Schröder et al. Screening and Prostate-Cancer Mortality in a Randomized European Study. N Engl J Med 2009;360:1310-9.

The second reason is the damage caused by the treatment, which many argue, especially in older men, is worse than the disease. The two commonest forms of treatment are surgery and radiotherapy. Surgery, as in total prostatectomy, is associated with a high incidence of permanent impotence (loss of normal sexual function) and hopefully transient, urinary incontinence. Radiotherapy is associated with a high risk of damaging the anal sphincter resulting in faecal incontinence, and not many older men enjoy having to wear a nappy again at the end of their lives.

So, should we men have our prostate screened? I don't think we really know yet. It can be a terrible disease in younger men, and even though it is less common in this group, it is more likely to kill you if you get it at a younger age. Perhaps we should confine screening to ages fifty through seventy only; however, there are many published guidelines and a lot of ongoing debate by the "experts."

CERVICAL CANCER

Cervical cancer in women is the other major cancer for which screening is available in developed countries. The cervix sits as the opening on the bottom of the uterus or womb and infection of the skin cells in this area by a common wart virus (human papilloma virus HPV) causes most of the cancers here. Australian research has resulted in a vaccine for the common forms of the virus and is likely to significantly reduce the incidence of this disease. Unfortunately, there are too many other types of this virus to target all of them in the vaccine, and screening is still likely to need to continue. HPV infection is one of the commonest forms of sexually transmitted disease, and if a woman has not been sexually active, she is not at risk and does not need screening. Screening involves a "smear," where a doctor uses an instrument to scrape cells off the cervix, and examines them under a microscope to look for pre-cancerous or cancerous cells. The benefit seems to be predominantly in older women; however, some would argue if younger women enrol in a screening program, they are more likely to continue.

In a review of the UK screening program, cervical screening of a woman aged thirty-five to sixty-four reduced the risk of cervical cancer by 60 to 80 percent. The risk reduction in women aged twenty-five to thirty-four years is described as "more modest." There is no question, however, that cervical cancer screening reduces the chance of dying from this disease and if it is available to you, it seems unwise not to participate in this type of screening.

Peter Sasieni et al. Effectiveness of cervical screening with age: population based case-control study of prospectively recorded data. BMJ. 2009; 339: b2968. Published online 2009 July 28. doi: 10.1136/bmj.b2968

ESOPHAGEAL CANCER

Cancer of the esophagus or gullet is not something routinely screened for but is worthy of special mention, as its precursor, Barrett's Esophagus, is associated with the metabolic syndrome. This has been linked to type 2 diabetes, independent of obesity, and to truncal obesity alone. Barrett's esophagus is a change in the cell type that lines the esophagus and occurs in response to reflux of fluid from the stomach back into the esophagus. Esophageal reflux causes the symptom heartburn.

These cells change from skin cells, like the skin on your arm, to cells like stomach lining. In this new lining, there is a 30 to 125 times increased risk of adenocarcinoma of the esophagus, a type of esophageal cancer. Once you receive a diagnosis of this type of cancer, your chance of being alive in five years is only about 10 percent, even with surgery, radiotherapy, and chemotherapy.

About one in fifty people have this change in their esophagus, and if they have reflux disease, this rises to one in ten.

van Soest EM, Dieleman JP, Siersema PD, Sturkenboom MC, Kuipers EJ. Increasing incidence of Barrett's oesophagus in the general population. Gut 2005;54:1062-6.

The worrying thing about this cancer is its incidence has increased 600 percent in the last thirty years, and it continues to increase. The primary risk factor for this cancer is reflux symptoms, and if these occur on a daily basis your risk is eight times higher than average. If you are obese, with a BMI over 40, your risk increases seven times, and, if diabetic, it doubles. What happens if you multiply all these numbers together if you have diabetes, are obese, and suffer from reflux symptoms?

Kendal BJ et al Gastro-oesophageal reflux symptoms, oesophagitis and Barrett's Oesophagus in the general population. Journal of Gastroenterology and Hepatology Sept. 2011

If an endoscopic examination of the esophagus and stomach (gastroscopy) identifies you as having Barrett's esophagus, then we would usually recommend you have regular examinations every couple of years to ensure you are not developing precancerous changes.. This is much like a woman having a PAP smear for cervical cancer, where we look for changes in the cells before they become malignant or, in other words, become cancer. Once they are cancerous, it is often too late.

Recent studies suggest some medications, particularly statins, aspirin, and non-steroidal anti-inflammatory drugs (NSAIDs) may prevent the development of cancer within the area of Barrett's esophagus. In one study, either a statin or an NSAID reduced the risk by about 50 percent and both together by 75 percent. Low dose aspirin reduced the risk in a dose-dependent fashion but did not reach statistical significance. It is early days yet with this data, and I would not necessarily recommend taking these drugs if you have Barrett's esophagus alone, as the side effects might outweigh the benefits.

Kastelein F. Nonsteroidal anti-inflammatory drugs and statins have chemopreventative effects in patients with Barrett's esophagus Gastroenterology 2011 Dec; 141(6) :2000-8

The importance of sleep

Everyone knows that we all function better after a good nights' sleep. Beyond this, we understand very little about the mechanisms of sleep and why we need it—at just the right amount, not too much and not too little. Your brain has an inbuilt clock that tells you when you should be awake and asleep, the so-called circadian rhythm. This clock is set by the day/night cycle related to the earth turning to face the sun and to face away from it. The bright sunlight reduces the brain's production of the chemical melatonin during wakeful times and increases this during sleep times. This inbuilt sleep/wake cycle follows the day night cycle, and if you move to the other side of the world these internal and external cycles are out of sync and account for issues such as jet lag. Your internal circadian rhythm relatively rapidly resets to the local day/night cycle, however. It also explains why blind people may have a lot of difficulty setting their own circadian rhythm with subsequent sleep difficulty. The circadian rhythm, like most functions, seems to work less well as we get older, resulting in increasing sleep disturbance with age.

During sleep, there are also changes in hormone levels, such as an important hormone cortisol, and in body temperature, which falls by about a degree.

We do know that disturbance of sleep has very significant implications in many areas, affecting both the quality and quantity of your life. It seems that not only does your brain need time to recharge itself, perhaps to build up levels of transmitter compounds, but the whole of your body's physiological processes that keep you alive need to be recharged. Sleep disturbance seems to have widespread effects on the hormone systems in your body, your immune system, and your metabolism. An increased risk of both heart disease and type 2 diabetes can be linked to disturbed sleep.

If you don't get any sleep, you die. Animal models with rats easily show this, but it is not exactly ethical to repeat the same experiments with humans, where we assume the same applies.

Now, it is not simply a matter of getting enough sleep. Too much sleep or too little sleep both have significant health implications. To look at the risk of dying from any cause, picture a U-shaped graph, with time slept along the x or bottom axis and risk of death on the y or vertical axis. The bottom of the U is at seven hours sleep, and if you go to either side, you are more likely to die. This is probably a real effect, as multiple studies show it.

A Japanese study of almost 100,000 people aged forty to seventy-nine years and followed for 14.3 years, showed this effect well.

If a person slept four hours per night compared with those who slept seven hours per night, they were 2.3 times as likely to die from heart disease if they were female and 1.47 times as likely to die from non-heart related causes. Overall, the total risk of dying for either sex is 1.3 times. If they slept for ten or more hours, their risk of death from stroke, cardiovascular disease, and non-cardiovascular related death was one and a half to two times for both sexes. Sleep duration seemed to have an effect on cancer incidence as well. At least two other large studies show similar findings. An English study followed 10,000 public servants aged thirty-five to fifty-five for up to seventeen years. Sleeping less than five hours was associated with a risk of dying from cardiovascular disease of 2.4 times (a 240 percent increase) and sleeping more than nine hours was associated with a 2.1 fold increase for death from non-cardiovascular diseases.

Interestingly, stroke is again overrepresented as a cause of death in those having longer sleep duration.

Arthur S. Walters et al. Review of the Relationship of Restless Legs Syndrome and Periodic Limb Movements in Sleep to Hypertension, Heart Disease, and Stroke. SLEEP, Vol. 32, No. 3, 2009

JE Gangwisch et al. Sleep Duration as a Risk Factor for Diabetes Incidence in a Large US Sample. Sleep. 2007 December 1; 30(12): 1667–1673.

The association between sleep disturbance, obesity, and the metabolic syndrome is also interesting. There is a potential "chicken and egg" problem here because of something called obstructive sleep apnea (OSA), where increased body weight results in increased soft tissue in the airway, which "cuts off" when sleeping, resulting in disturbed sleep. The result is much less quality sleep time. We can argue that OSA is part of the metabolic syndrome in that it correlates better with waist/hip circumference and insulin resistance than it does with neck anatomy, such as a thick neck. Local surgery to "open" the airway is rarely successful; however, weight loss or gain does have significant effects on improving or worsening the syndrome.

Paul E. Peppard et al. Longitudinal Study of Moderate Weight Change and Sleep-Disordered Breathing. JAMA 2000; 284: 3015–21.

The association between OSA and insulin resistance or the metabolic syndrome is complex and poorly understood but may be independent of obesity. OSA itself is a huge problem for individuals and our society in general, with the resultant increase in daytime sleepiness resulting in increased traffic and work accidents. It is also strongly associated with hypertension, diabetes, and the polycystic ovarian syndrome, to mention a few. Short sleep duration independent of OSA and obesity is associated with insulin resistance and type 2 diabetes. Restricting healthy volunteers to four hours of sleep for six nights resulted in insulin resistance developing.

Karine Spiegel et al. Impact of sleep debt on metabolic and endocrine function. Lancet 1999; 354: 1435–39.

When it comes to obesity and sleep, which is what most of you are interested in, there is a relatively strong association between short sleep duration and weight gain or obesity. This effect is strongest in children and young adults and seems to wane with age. It would appear that it is the short sleep duration, which comes first and causes the obesity, rather than the obesity causing short sleep duration via OSA or another mechanism. In multiple studies, short sleep duration in children is strongly associated with current and future obesity (five out of five prospective studies). Similar results were found in young adults (seventeen out of twenty-three studies reviewed)

J C K Wells et al. Sleep patterns and television viewing in relation to obesity and blood pressure: evidence from an adolescent Brazilian birth cohort. International Journal of Obesity (2008) 32, 1042–1049; doi:10.1038/ijo.2008.37; published online 18 March 2008

Both animal studies and human studies show that experimentally restricting sleep results in increased appetite and increased calorie intake. The increased appetite seems to be particularly for high-fat and high-carbohydrate foods. These changes correlated with changes in the levels of chemicals in the blood stream, which control hunger (increased ghrelin, decreased leptin).

Jeffrey S. Flier. A Good Night's Sleep: Future Antidote to the Obesity Epidemic? Ann Intern Med December 7, 2004 141:885-886

Shahrad Taheri et al. Short Sleep Duration Is Associated with Reduced Leptin, Elevated Ghrelin, and Increased Body Mass Index. December 2004 Issue of PLoS Medicine

A number of studies show this. The other obvious issue is if you are awake longer, you have more time to eat, especially if you are sitting watching TV.

Chronic sleep deprivation also leads to fatigue, which itself is likely to result in reduced physical activity when awake. Some studies associate short sleep duration with reduced participation in physical activity and increased TV watching.

Sleep may also play a part in thermoregulation with sleep deprivation shown to cause a drop in core body temperature in several studies. This results in a drop in metabolic rate and in fuel consumed, with the residual fuel available to turn into fat, to store for that "rainy day" that may never come.

PJ Shaw, Thermoregulatory changes. Basic Science, Physiology, and Behavior. Marcel Dekker: New York, 2005, pp 319–338.

Emotional well-being: what we think and feel, does it matter if we are unhappy?

Many studies in the literature show that if you are happy you are more likely to be successful in many areas not only related to your health, but also your friendships, work performance, marriage, and financial income. We are only interested in the health implication here; however, as you can see, there are many other benefits from simply feeling good about yourself and your life.

There is evidence to suggest an association between being happy and longevity; however, most of the studies in the literature look at things the other way around, showing that a negative attitude or depressed mood are associated with a shorter lifespan and more disease. A person's mood is clearly not like counting the number of cards in a pack, it is a rather soft and fuzzy entity difficult to quantify, and various psychological tests designed to measure it are far from perfect. We need to keep this in mind when assessing the studies

The Cardiovascular Health Study is a large population-based study that followed 5201 American men and women over sixty-five years of age living in the community. The authors controlled for (in other words, tried to take out the effect of) other factors such as socioeconomic class, other medical diseases, and behavioral factors, such as smoking or lack of exercise. Over six years of follow up 984 of the participants died. High depressive score rating was an independent risk factor for dying, with an increased risk of 25 percent when compared to those with low depressive scores. If we just look at depression alone without trying to control for other factors as above, the increased risk was 43 percent.

Richard Schulz et al. Association Between Depression and Mortality in Older Adults The Cardiovascular Health Study. Arch Intern Med. 2000;160:1761-1768

In the group described above the author postulated the increased mortality in depression was associated with cardiovascular disease. Certainly, studies have linked depressive symptoms, such as fatigue to a higher risk of having a heart attack.

A.Appels et al. Excess fatigue as a precursor of myocardial infarction. Heart J 9:758–764, 1988

There is, however, evidence linking depression to other serious diseases such as type 2 diabetes. Another study followed 11,615 non-diabetic community-based adults, aged forty-eight to sixty-seven, for six years looking for the development of type 2 diabetes. They assessed depression by scoring fatigue, sleep disturbance, feelings of hopelessness, loss of libido, and increased irritability. Those with the highest scores of depression had a 63 percent increased risk of developing diabetes when compared to those with the lowest scores. When they attempted to control or 'take out' the effect of other factors, such as smoking, physical inactivity, blood pressure, diet, and obesity, there was still a 38 percent increased risk. They postulate this may relate to changes in the levels of some hormones in the blood stream, such as cortisol and catecholamines, which rise in depression and inhibit the effect of insulin.

Briana Mezuk. Depression and Type 2 Diabetes Over the Lifespan. A meta-analysis. Diabetes Care December 2008 vol. 31 no. 12 2383-2390

So, accepting that depression is associated with a higher risk of dying overall and, in particular, a higher risk of heart disease and diabetes, the next question is, why should this be the case?

Clearly, depression may result in unhealthy behavior, such as cigarette smoking and lack of physical activity. Attempts to control for these things in studies may be inadequate.

There is also the possibility that depression has an effect on the body's inbuilt functions, including the immune system, hormones, inflammation, the nervous system, or other systems we have not considered. These effects may cause a higher rate of some diseases and shorter lifespan. A recent article shows depression has been linked to raised inflammatory markers (CRP), changes in hormone levels (catecholamines and cortisol), and loss of immune response to vaccination.

A study involving 216 men and women looked at some of these factors, graded them from one to five on happiness scores, and found a number of differences. The level of the stress hormone cortisol, released from the adrenal gland, was significantly higher in those with lower happiness scores. There was no significant difference in blood pressure.

A blood clotting factor, fibrinogen, was shown to be released in a significantly higher amount, after stress, in those with lower levels of happiness scoring, when compared to those with higher levels of happiness scoring. This ratio was twelve times higher in those with lowest versus highest happiness scores.

The level of fibrinogen in the plasma is a predictor of future heart disease increasing the risk of atheroma and clots, and this may be part of the explanation relating to the relationship between depression and increased mortality.

Andrew Steptoe et al. Positive affect and health-related neuroendocrine, cardiovascular, and inflammatory processes. PNAS May 3, 2005 vol. 102 no. 18 6508-6512

CHAPTER 3

Why Do We Age? Why do We Need to Die?

CLIMATE CHANGE MAY be topical at present but is in no way a new phenomenon; it has been going on since life began. Currently, however, the main argument is about whom to blame.

The world is a constantly changing place, and to survive, organisms large and small must constantly adapt to have the best chance of survival in their new environment. Those that do not adapt are more likely to die, and this probability of survival or lack of survival is the basis of evolution. The best adapted are more likely to survive, and if you play this scenario over hundreds or thousands of times, as evolution does, they are the only ones to survive.

Each time we produce a new generation, the offspring are not the same as their parents. As you are all well aware, everyone is an individual with different physical and emotional traits. Differences include traits, such as red hair and fair skin or darker hair and darker skin, as is the case in two of my own sons. These physical and emotional differences make the offspring more or less likely to survive in a harsh environment. In our modern world, we could argue that evolution has ceased, as the harsh environment that shapes it no longer exists. Survival of the fittest is no longer the case.

A good example of evolution is black or white skin in humans. Archeologists believe all humans to have come out of Africa and to have been black skinned at that time. Those who migrated to cold climates, such as Europe, very quickly lost their pigmentation. Scientists speculate this happened within a few thousand years—very quickly in evolutionary terms. The evolutionary pressure here is likely to have been vitamin D, this is made in the skin from sunlight, and if you are black, living in an area with very little sunlight, you quickly become deficient. As previously discussed, vitamin D's role in the body is very complicated, and we are only just coming to grips with some of the details. We have known for years it is important in calcium absorption and bone strength, but it also is very important in immune function. Studies suggest that very low levels, for example, may make you up to eight times more likely to die from infections such as tuberculosis when compared to people with high levels. This is just one example of why a person with dark skin may have been much more likely to die than one with fair skin in early Europe, it is likely there will have been many others. The result is obviously that the fairer your skin the more likely you are to survive, which implies to breed and produce more fair skinned offspring, something reinforced again and again with each generation. Any dark-skinned individuals who survived by chance would have mated with fair-skinned individuals, and their genes for dark skin would have diluted out.

So what does this all have to do with aging and life expectancy?

Well, the only chance evolution gets to change or adapt a species is with each new generation, on which it then exerts survival pressures. If a species lives a very long time before it breeds it will not be able to adapt and will become extinct. Ideally, a species should breed as frequently as possible to allow it to change and adapt with a short time between generations, making survival more likely.

This is why tiny organisms such as bacteria, which go through life cycles very quickly in our terms, are so quick to adapt to new environmental threats, such as developing resistance to new antibiotics. Some of the bacteria, which "accidentally" develop drug resistance, such as not letting the drug get through their cell membranes, survive; the others die. All the surviving bacteria then have drug resistance. This happens in hours to days. Large animals however, such as woolly mammoths, which were roaming the earth ten thousand years ago during the ice age, could not cope with climate change evolving over a few thousand years. There are none left today.

So why do we have to die off after we breed? Well, unfortunately, if we all lived for a thousand years, there would not be enough food or resources to go around, and we would be a burden to our offspring, making them less likely to survive and to breed; therefore, this group or species would be more likely to die off too.

The optimal, in terms of evolution, is to die as soon as possible after producing and raising offspring, unless living just a bit longer may have survival advantages for the next generation. This is perhaps the case in humans, where grandparents may have helped care for the very young, for example, while parents went off to hunt.

In other words, your mortality and death are of survival advantage for your species, and the pressures of evolution have shaped the potential length of your life. We do this by ageing, or better put, "getting old and falling to bits," as my father would say.
This necessity of ageing and dying is programmed into our genes and something over which we have had no control. Well, up to now anyway. We are just beginning to understand the way our genes do control the length of our lives, and it is very likely that within the not–too-distant future we will start interfering with these processes and have artificially longer lives. Researchers in this area have recently said that we may be the last generation to have a "natural" life expectancy.

CHAPTER 4

Recommendations for a Long and Healthy Life

THIS IS ESSENTIALLY a summary of the contents of the book and, if you are in a hurry, perhaps the only part you need to read.

It should be clear to you from reading this book that one of the major changes in modern society is the amount of exercise we have to do to simply exist. Evolution has not had time to adapt us to this new environment, as in evolutionary terms, it has come upon us instantaneously—a bit like a comet striking the earth in the dinosaur times. Where are all the dinosaurs now? Where are we headed?

I am of course excluding our current efforts to imitate the dinosaurs in asking this question. Human beings pretending to be dinosaurs don't count.

Because of this relative lack of exercise, and in part related to dietary changes, this evil monster, the metabolic syndrome, has fallen upon us. You don't have to be a genius to see how to reverse this situation, do you? We are much more fortunate than the dinosaurs. At least we know what we need to do.

This is not about an exercise program, a new fad diet, or a short-term goal to reduce your weight by 10 kg. We know that when obese people go on diets, no matter how determined they are, about 95 percent of them will fail to maintain the weight loss by two years. They will have achieved their pre-diet weight, or in other words, achieved nothing.

If you want to succeed, you have to look at your life and current habits in their entirety and make a major *lifestyle* change. In other words, you need to look at everything you do from the moment you get up in the morning until you go to bed, and think about how you can change it permanently for a better outcome. What can you do differently? If you do not do this, you *will* fail. You have to be committed to succeed and committed in the long-term. There is no going back to your old habits. This is arguably the most important message in the whole book. Please stop reading and take a moment to consider how it applies to you.

No one ever plans to fail, but most people fail to plan.

Exercise

Exercise is, I think, the most important of the changes; however, they all need to occur simultaneously. You will have to look at how to incorporate this into your lifestyle. Any exercise is good; however, up to a point, the more the better. Having to run in front of a rickshaw for fourteen hours per day is enough to damage your heart; however, I doubt any of you will be able to achieve this.

Ideally, include forty-five minutes or more a day of raising your heart rate to at least 70 percent of your predicted safe maximum. Remember your safe maximum is roughly 220 minus your age, and you should take it slowly to begin with if you have been a practicing couch potato over recent months—it is only a guide. This type of aerobic exercise is probably the safest and the best to begin with.

Can you ride a bicycle to work? Preferably, on a bike path if available, as a bus is less likely to run you down.

Do you really need to drive your car to work? What about briskly walking to the nearest bus or train if you cannot ride a bike—helping the environment at the same time?

Can you go for a brisk walk up a local hill or a jog if your joints are up to it before or after work? Can you do swimming training in the local pool? No, your sore knee does not qualify as an excuse here. What sports are available in the community that you could participate in?

If you cannot imagine life without TV or a computer, or it is not safe to go outside, then you will just have to put your exercise bike or jogging machine in front of the TV/computer and ditch the couch, or at least move it to the side.

I cannot do this for you, including *thinking* of options relevant to you. You will have to use your brain as well as your body. I am only giving a few suggestions. You may not find any of this brief list applicable to you; however, I am sure you can think of something you can do or change.

Personal trainers generally say you should have a day off a week to let your body recover. You know what I think of "expert opinions" and I am not aware of any evidence to support this but would happily accept it if you are more likely to comply with the new exercise regime you have incorporated into your new lifestyle.

Save your list of excuses for not exercising for your gravestone, I'm not interested. Remember you will be a long time dead.

Diet and Weight loss

Diet, exercise, or preferably both will reverse the metabolic syndrome. The problem is that dieting alone does not achieve sustainable weight loss in our society; you need to do more than just diet to keep the weight off, and you need to keep doing it.

The hidden enemy here is carbohydrate. Food manufacturers sneak it into almost everything they make. Their aim is to make food and drink taste good so you will buy it and they will make money, very simple. They are not the slightest bit concerned with your health. That is your problem! Perhaps if we made your health their concern we would get some changes at a community level, but this is clearly not likely to happen in the short term in your lifetime. Personally, I favor heavily taxing unhealthy food, as this is likely to be the most effective approach to changing habits at a societal level. No government seems to have the courage or backbone to do this, unfortunately, but the time may come.

You need to start taking responsibility for yourself and your family and interpreting food manufacturer's messages accurately. For example, "low in fat" usually means, "loaded with sugar." Try reading how much sugar (carbohydrate) there is in your low-fat strawberry yogurt. There is a reason it tastes so good. If you feel good about eating it then the kindest label I have for you is ignorant. The same is true of most processed breakfast cereals. If they say "low in fat," they are likely at least 20 to 30 percent sugar. For "toasted" muesli, you should read, "deep fried in the cheapest and least healthy oil available" and "loaded with sugar." Probably goes well with your "low fat" yogurt. What a good start to the day!

The American approach of having a donut with coffee for rushed breakfast is another good example. A donut is processed white flour, fried in toxic oil (to your heart and blood vessels that is, let alone its carcinogenic, cancer-causing potential) and then rolled in sugar. No wonder it tastes so good! Thank goodness, you had a cup of coffee full of antioxidants to protect you from some of the donut issues. Or did you say you had soft drink with it? Oh well, that is only about thirteen teaspoons or sugar per can, but at least it is low in fat!

Now, you might think this is all starting to sound a bit extreme or ridiculous; however, this is what most of you do every day of your lives and I am only scratching the surface. Should I move on to analyze lunch at the fast-food outlet you were visiting?

So, do you want to leave responsibility for your dietary intake to the "conscience" of the processed food manufacturers, or do you want to take control yourself?

The take-home message to remember here is unless you critically read exactly what is in processed foods, *don't eat processed foods.*

This does include things as simple as toasted muesli and low-fat fruit yogurt. I never said this was going to be easy and not require effort on your part, did I?

What is wrong with fresh fruit, vegetables, meat, fish, poultry, grains, lentils, breads, and dairy products, including unsweetened, low-fat dairy just to list a few of your options.

There are healthy processed foods out there; you just need to read the labels and think before you buy if you are going to eat processed foods.

Do I really need to say anything about fast foods loaded with fat, salt and sugar? Why don't you do some homework here; the internet is a powerful tool. I can virtually guarantee you will be shocked at what you find out.

In terms of what sort of unprocessed foods to eat I want to keep things simple, you can look at the details earlier in the book if you wish, but the age-old saying of everything in moderation is still reasonable, especially if you are going to make up for any dietary indiscretions with extra exercise.

In general terms, however, avoid red meat and focus on eating poultry and fish. Excluding health issues, there are emotional and environmental reasons for considering this. Do you really like the idea of eating relatively intelligent mammals? Would you be happy eating your dog or cat? Perhaps you could use these types of thoughts to steer you away from red meat at an emotional level.

At an environmental level, it is worth knowing it takes fewer limited resources to make a serving of fish or chicken than a serving of beef or lamb. So, when you have the fish or chicken you could argue you are doing your bit to save the planet. Regarding plant protein, it takes ten times as much arable land to make a kilogram of beef compared to a kilogram of plant protein. I would not recommend becoming an absolute vegetarian, however, because you really need to know what you are doing if you are to avoid protein malnutrition. That is not to say that lentil or soy burgers are not a good option from time to time on health, emotional, and environmental grounds.

Remember protein may be useful in helping with weight loss, as it tends to cause satiety or a feeling of being satisfied, reducing your appetite more than carbohydrate or fat. Eat the fish first and then pause and have a chat, to allow yourself to feel "full" before moving on to the chips, or if possible, avoiding them altogether. Do not forget, the only guaranteed way of losing weight is through reduced calorific intake, and the last thing you really need is the chips.

Where fats and oils are concerned, remember they contain a lot of calories but are probably not as bad as we have been led to believe in the last thirty years. If possible, avoid animal fats, but not at the expense of using adulterated vegetable fats such as trans-fatty acids. In other words, the butter may not be as bad for you as the margarine, and the 100-percent vegetable oil that your fish and chips was fried in may be very bad for you, as it is likely all trans-fatty acid. Try to focus on polyunsaturated and monounsaturated fats such as olive oil, which we think do convey health benefits. If you really must fry something, use rice bran or peanut oil, both of which are relatively heat stable.

Where fruit and vegetables are concerned, if they taste very sweet it is because they contain a lot of sugar. This type of sugar is just as bad for you as processed sugar, which is simply purified from sugar cane and is called sucrose. Fructose is the sugar in fruit and honey and more readily turns into fat in the liver, possibly making it worse than sucrose. It is very sweet, something food manufacturers have noted for years, and they are putting fructose in your soft drinks and candies to get you to buy more of them. They have no interest in your liver, only your wallet. Having said this, I am simply making the point, again, that because you feel something is natural or comes from fruit does not necessarily make it good for you, especially in large amounts. All fruits and vegetables contain good antioxidants, especially the brightly colored ones, so go for those if possible. Within reason, do not go overboard with consumption of very sweet fruits or vegetables, for example mangoes and beetroot.

Dietary Supplements

Where vitamins are concerned, the only one I would consider taking myself is vitamin D. The level-one evidence is not yet there to be dogmatic about this for "general health" benefits outside of deficiency states; however, circumstantial evidence is, I think, strong. Coupled with this, it is relatively non-toxic, and even if you do not do yourself any good you are unlikely to do any harm. I would recommend doses higher than generally advised at 3000 to 5000 IU per day and then getting your doctor to check your serum vitamin D level in three to six months to check you are not outside the normal range. Aim for the "high normal" range on blood testing. I have been taking 3000 to 5000 IU daily for two years and still have a level that is only high normal.

The evidence for taking other vitamins at high levels is even less strong, except perhaps with respect to folic acid if you are pregnant. Low folic acid level is associated with fetal malformations, and supplementation prevents these.

Mega dose vitamin B does nothing for common colds or hangovers but is very good at turning your urine bright yellow if you are into that sort of thing. It probably does not do you any harm (as far as we know), but it is only in your blood stream for an hour or two before you pee it out.

Be careful with mineral supplements because many of these are potentially very toxic, especially the trace element minerals.

Calcium supplements have been recommended for decades to preserve bone strength; however, if you are getting adequate intake in your diet there is no evidence they work and there is some evidence they may do harm by calcifying your blood vessels and increasing your risk for vascular disease, such as heart attacks.

Magnesium is probably relatively harmless if your kidneys work normally and is good at stabilizing electrical activity in cell membranes, so may help prevent cardiac arrhythmias and muscle cramps. It is not unreasonable to take this in an absorbable form, such as magnesium aspartate at a dose of 1 to 2 grams per day. If you take non-absorbable magnesium, such as magnesium sulphate or Epsom salts, they will go straight through you, literally.

Iron supplementation is dangerous unless you are deficient. Sorting out if you are deficient is a simple blood test from your doctor. Iron supplementation is likely to make you feel much better if you do need it. It is freely available; however, only take one or, at maximum, two of the tablets daily if you are advised to take it.

Zinc is important for immune function and as mentioned does seem to change the outcome in gut and chest infections, possibly including the common cold. Dietary supplementation would be reasonable with zinc sulphate at 50 to 100 mg daily. Beware this may cause copper deficiency, and if you are planning to take it for years, get your serum copper and zinc checked after twelve months.

With the exception of zinc, taking other trace elements for health reasons without medical supervision is dangerous.

Other foods

In this section of the book, I summarize some of the properties of a number of common foods that may confer health benefits outside their basic nutritional value. This is by no means a complete list; however, you should consider taking some or all of these on a regular basis. If possible, take in a small amount every day but not if this interferes with other aims such as weight loss. This is in addition to your diet rich in fresh fruit and vegetables as described previously.

These include:

Dark chocolate

Coffee

Green tea

Red wine (no more than two glasses per day)

Olive oil

Fish oil, preferably from cold seas

Tree nuts

RECOMMENDED CONVENTIONAL MEDICATION FOR OVER FORTY- TO FIFTY-YEAR-OLDS:

Aspirin

I've summarized the evidence to support this and the potential for harm in the text. It is very complex. In the past, we have tried to balance the reduced risk of vascular events, such as heart attacks and thrombotic (clot caused) strokes with the increased risk for bleeding, be it from ulcers caused in the stomach, bleeding into the brain as in a hemorrhagic stroke, or bleeding following trauma from a motor vehicle or sports injury, for example.

The medical profession has never really considered the issue of cancer prevention in the assessment of aspirin's good and bad points, and there seems little doubt that aspirin may be helpful in reducing the risk of many of the more common cancers. The evidence is relatively neutral at this time in terms of conveying survival advantage or reducing your overall risk of dying. This may be because you are more likely to die from a bleeding ulcer and less likely to die from a heart attack; however, it may also be we do not have the data to analyze yet, to enable us to draw sensible conclusions.

On balance I think taking regular aspirin is a good idea; however, as cancer prevention is one of the aims, a person does need to take a higher dose for this effect (600 mg) than for that to reduce the risk of vascular disease(75 mg). The big risk is bleeding from ulcers. If you are already on a drug to control ulcers or reflux disease, such as a proton-pump inhibitor, your risk of life threatening bleeding is greatly reduced, and there is no question in my mind that you should be taking aspirin. I would suggest 600 mg daily. If you are on no other medication, only take aspirin at this dose under medical supervision and regular review, including risk discussion with your doctor.

Antihypertensives (ACE inhibitors, ARBs)

See text for the details relating to these drug types.

As previously discussed, what constitutes normal blood pressure is the issue, and well within the normal range there is evidence that high normal conveys a significantly increased risk of stroke and heart attack than low normal does. In an ideal world, I would define high blood pressure as a systolic pressure over 115 mm Hg, which I expect most of my colleagues will consider too low. The problem is any higher puts you at increased risk and, as the above drugs seem to have health benefits outside simply controlling blood pressure, I would consider starting on a low dose at systolic blood pressure of 115 mm Hg, especially once you are over forty years of age. The down side is who is going to pay for the medication? Because the risk reduction is small, as is the individual cost (less than a cup of coffee), I think it should be the patient not the health care system.

The statins

These cholesterol-lowering tablets seem to convey other health benefits, outside of lowering cholesterol levels. There is a small risk of harm from liver and muscle inflammation; however, I consider the benefits outweigh the risks and around the age of fifty a person should consider taking a small dose, for example atorvastatin at 20 mg daily. This is especially true if you are a male at higher risk for vascular disease and prostate cancer. The same issues relating to cost apply.

Screening for common cancers

If your health-care service offers screening programs for cancers it is because they can afford the substantial cost and because they feel the risk of the screening is outweighed by the benefit of finding early (potentially curable) cancers. You would have to have rocks in your head not to participate in these programs. The only common cancers routinely screened for at present are bowel, breast, and cervical cancer. Read the section in the book again and make an informed decision as to the absolute risk reduction and the most effective form of screening, particularly where bowel cancer is concerned.

Sleep

As already discussed, you should be aiming for six to eight hours of sleep per night, ideally seven. It is easy to ensure you do not get too much sleep with the numerous devices we have at our disposal to wake us up.

The problem most of us have is getting enough sleep and especially quality sleep. Lying awake in bed all night does not count. If you search the internet for helpful hints to get to sleep and to sleep well, you are likely to find useful information in a very short time, relative to the time you may spend lying awake in your bed trying to get to sleep.

Useful hints include:

Avoid caffeine for six hours before going to bed
Not eating for three hours and avoid drinking for two hours before bed
Avoid drinking excessive alcohol in the evening
Read or listen to relaxing music before sleeping
Rise early
Exercise regularly to improve sleep quality
Sleep in a darkened room

Sleep in a separate room from you partner if you continually wake each other up.

Practice relaxation exercises, such as deep breathing. Visualize in your mind a relaxed environment and the feeling of tiredness.

Use tricks to stop focusing on all the stressors of the day, or worrying about tomorrow. For example, it is very difficult to think about these things if you visualize in your mind actually drawing numbers beginning at one hundred, circling them with a pen, and counting slowly down, one by one, especially if you are a man!

This list could go on forever, you just have to try to find out what works for you. If all else fails, take melatonin before bed, preferably a slow-release formulation.

Happiness

Humankind has been seeking the answer to this question for as long as we have existed. We could spend the rest of our lives reading the extensive literature on this topic.

Clearly, we do not have all the answers; however, there are a few simple things you can practice in your life that may help. If you succeed, you will live a longer and happier life.

Happiness is clearly a state of mind related to various chemical levels in the brain. These chemical levels and your perception of happiness fluctuate every minute of every day of your life. Some things that may help to maximize these include:

Keep reminding yourself of the things you have not the things you do not have. Simple things you take for granted such as your eyesight, your ability to walk, to talk, relationships... Would you rather own a Porsche or have the gift of vision? Just remind yourself how lucky you really are! I wouldn't give up my eyesight for any amount of money or material wealth.

Seek out friends and new relationships, and value those you already have. It is your interaction with other people, not material goods, that will convey long-lasting happiness.

Forgive and don't dwell on negative interactions with others. Those friends are precious.

Have a purpose to strive for in life. If you do not have one then think of one! Caring for others or aiming to make others happy is a good option, as it appears to have dramatic effects on your own level of happiness.

Exercise regularly—funny how this keeps raising its head! Exercise increases the levels of several chemicals in the brain that are associated with improved mood in the short term but also seems to correlate with happier people in the longer term, quite apart from curing the metabolic syndrome.

Have a spiritual or religious belief; if you can achieve this good on you, some of us cannot achieve this.

Enjoy regular sexual intercourse with more than three orgasms per week, which correlates with happiness and longevity, so get to it!

In brief, learn to be an optimist not a pessimist.

"A pessimist sees difficulty in every opportunity; an optimist sees opportunity in every difficulty," is one of Winston Churchill's most famous quotes. How do you see the messages in this book?

CONCLUSION

I would like to give you a couple of things to think about in summing up the messages in this book, relating to the way you look at your life and your personal motivation to do something about the issues at hand. Close friends suggested the examples below. I hope that you can think back to them in the future during 'times of need' when your motivation wanes.

Imagine you are out shopping, and as you are a bit bored, you buy yourself a brand new parachute to play with. You then go to the top of a large skyscraper of more than one hundred stories and leap off the roof.

You have the sensation you are flying through the air, just like Superman, completely relaxed, weightless, and content in free fall toward the ground.

As you sail past the twentieth floor, someone sticks his head out the window and says, "Hey, mate, don't you think you should pull the cord on your parachute now?"

You reply, "Why? Nothing is wrong! I'm having a great time! It doesn't look like I needed to bring the chute after all."

Does this example describe your passage through life?

Which floor are you currently "sailing past"? How close are you to the ground? Are you living in a state of denial?

There will come a time when it is too late to pull the cord; however, if you are reading this book it is unlikely you are there yet.

Once you are dead or severely maimed, that is it. You will not get a second chance to pull that parachute cord, or to change your habits. A stroke, heart attack, and death are one-way events; you cannot go back and undo them once they occur.

You do not think this applies to you?

Well, try visiting the hospital wards and see how many people your age or slightly older are lying there having had strokes, heart attacks, or having developed various cancers. They did not think it applied to them either! They are arguably the lucky ones; the others are lying in graveyards with no chance to reflect on what might have been if they had "pulled the cord" a few years ago and changed their lifestyle.

A sobering and insightful comment from another friend says this: "When the student is ready the teacher appears."

Sure, he has a very good point; however, I am hoping that reading this short book has moved you slightly closer to the "ready" stage. Are you "ready" to make changes?

To put things another way, let me quote the title of another book, about another topic, but which I think sums these things up nicely:

"If you want to walk on water, *you've got to get out of the boat!*"

Yes, I do think you can walk on water. You just have to put your mind to it.

So, stop talking about it and get out of the bloody boat!

www.ingramcontent.com/pod-product-compliance
Lightning Source LLC
Chambersburg PA
CBHW070138290526
45789CB00002B/530